"Maya Hennessey is an incredibly energetic, motivated, and ⟨expert. Her warmth and understanding weave through every ⟨word, ⟩ participants on a walk through her life and her soul—passing on to others the healing techniques that she has discovered throughout her personal and professional journey."

Linda Henderson
Prevention Resource Development Project
Prevent Child Abuse Illinois

"Maya's charisma and her engaging style are the marks of an outstanding presenter and workshop leader, as her expertise and passion for oppressed women keep weaving their way throughout the addictions field."

Bill L. White
Author, *Slaying the Dragon: The History of Addiction and Treatment and Recovery in America.*
Evaluator Project SAFE (1986-2002)

"Maya's presentations are heartfelt and refreshing, as she shares her life experiences, while offering invaluable techniques to help us better serve our customers."

Annie Griffin
Rehabilitation Services Supervisor
State of Illinois Department of Human Services

"As a trainer Maya Hennessey combines two traits perfectly: warmth and knowledge. With her warmth she brings the room into her circle, and with her knowledge she delivers complex concepts into easily assimilated experiential skills and techniques."

Joe Rosenfeld, Ph.D
Curriculum and Training Coordinator
Great Lakes Addiction Technology Transfer Center

"Maya Hennessey is one of the nation's most compassionate speakers, offering comfort and solutions to the afflicted and their helpers."

Mark Sanders
CEO / Author / Trainer
On The Mark Consulting

If Only I'd Had This Caregiving Book

Maya Hennessey

EMAIL:MAYAHENNESSEY@SBCGLOBAL.NET ◆ WEBSITE:WWW.MAYAHENNESSEY.COM

Bloomington, IN

authorHOUSE

Milton Keynes, UK

AuthorHouse™
1663 Liberty Drive, Suite 200
Bloomington, IN 47403
www.authorhouse.com
Phone: 1-800-839-8640

AuthorHouse™ UK Ltd.
500 Avebury Boulevard
Central Milton Keynes, MK9 2BE
www.authorhouse.co.uk
Phone: 08001974150

First published by AuthorHouse 01/03/06

ISBN: 1-4259-1299-0 (e)
ISBN: 1-4259-0974-4 (sc)

Library of Congress Control Number: 2005911096

Printed in the United States of America
Bloomington, Indiana

This book is printed on acid-free paper.

Acknowledgments

Lonetta Albright, Rick Alonzo, Jane Brown-Mardsen, Mike Bruni, Sherrie Brutskus, Ben Coblenz, Theresa Colvin, Ruth Cung, Lorie Donovan, Bob Carty, Cancer Wellness Center in Northbrook, Illinois, Kathleen and Chuck Chapman, Deann Dusek, Family Learning Center in South Bend, Indiana, Jill Friedman, Loreli Golden, Jamella Goosby, Yolanda Green, Laurie Graciana, Annie Griffin, Clara Harrington, Linda Henderson, Bruce Joleaud, Jean Knoll, Roger Krause, Sandy Lipton, Jim Long, Sharon McCarthy—Hospice, Cathy McNeilly, Lynne Malnekopf, Phyllis Marder, Hal Mead, Susan Miller, Oasis, Brian Pacwa, Dawn Paskowitz, Mike Peters, Renee Popovits, Molly Redenbaugh, Brian Rooney, Joe Rosenfeld, Peg Ryder, Susan Moses, Mark Sanders, Chuck Skelton, Bill White , Melanie Whitter, LaDonna Williams, and all my friends at the State of Illinois Division of Alcoholism and Substance Abuse are gratefully acknowledged for all of their help and support.

My deepest appreciation to Brian Rooney for generously sharing his dissertation. Just reading it gave me hope and opened my mind to the possibility that I could mobilize, organize, and coordinate the help I needed. Thanks also for patiently listening to my tears and heartache. I wouldn't have survived my caregiving ordeal without Brian.

My deep appreciation goes out to my two closest friends—Deann and Lynne, whose listening, loving, and unconditional acceptance sustained then and still does.

My appreciation also goes out to phantom neighbors who did all the lawn care, and to all the people who advocated for me and defended me when I wasn't present to defend myself. And those of you whose names and/or kindnesses I can't recall right now, please know that the impact of your compassion left its mark and made my life easier. God, as you understand him, knows your kindnesses. Should you have a need, I pray that God's angels will appear for you, as you did for me.

Both a disclaimer and a tremendous appreciation go out to all those whose books, workshops, and ideas have shaped and formed me, even if today I can't recall their names or the titles of their books. My appreciation goes to the thousands of teachers, mentors, authors, and workshop leaders, who taught me well, and whose rich creativity worked its way into my psyche, and then out into the world in the form of my workshops and the exercises I created, which others give me credit for, but wouldn't exist without your creativity and influence.

My most tender appreciation goes to all the caregivers who shared their stories, whose names I changed, as promised. And for all caregivers past, present, and future.

Table of Contents

IF ONLY I'D HAD THIS CAREGIVING BOOK
Maya Hennessey

Introduction and How to Use This Book

INTRODUCING THE CAREGIVER'S MODEL

My late husband and I had lots of friends, with varied skills and resources, eager to help. Yet I was nearly destroyed by my vicious "To-Do" List, until I started applying the principles that you'll be introduced to in this book. Later on, I adapted the exercises so all caregivers could weave my model through their unique situations and personalities.

When you are called—perhaps suddenly!—by fate and circumstance to be the one ultimately responsible for care and daily living needs of another person, please know that you are not alone. Family members, friends, and various agencies are approachable, helpful, and often eager to help you in managing the burdens of caregiving.

This book helps guide you through the process of analyzing your needs as a caregiver, guiding you through a process that will sustain you through it all.

The premise stands that each caregiver is unique, and each will find different aspects of the model beneficial. You have been given a call to duty, and this book was crafted to help you answer that call, whatever the circumstances involved.

HOW TO PROCEED

To get the most from this book, go through it from start to finish, completing all the exercises and highlighting those sections that affect you specifically. Then, because your caregiving routine is always evolving and demands continual shifting, feel free to repeat the exercises you found most meaningful. You'll likely notice different results each time you revisit an exercise.

This book results from my own caregiving experience. I discovered the benefits of developing a model that was adaptable to the ever-changing demands of caregiving. Friends soon took to calling the whole process "Maya's Model," and, with humble thanks to them and for ease of reference to the collective particulars, so it will be called throughout the book.

The Model consists of three interwoven components (1) You, (2) Your To-Do List, (3) Your Social Support Network. As the exercises strengthen the components, you'll find they have a steadying effect, and you are better able to fulfill the role of caregiving.

CHAPTERS

Chapter 1 is my story of caregiving. I share my steady physical, mental, attitudinal, situational, and constitutional deterioration as I tried to keep rising up to the mounting impossible demands as my dying husband's principal caregiver; the mistakes I made; and lessons I learned, some applied too late. Chapter 2 is an overview and sampling of Maya's Model. Chapters 3 through 8 delve deeper into each of the components, with exercises to evoke insight, strategies, and personal power to reduce the stress of caregiving. As the exercises in this book keep strengthening each of the components, you'll feel the benefits of thriving and surviving, growing in absolute certainty that it can keep you afloat come what may.

Keep a notebook, a journal, to record your answers to the exercises, and journal/write about the feelings and insights that come up as you proceed through the book. Studies show that journaling (writing about your feelings) eases distress and increases awareness of solutions. Record your answers and reactions in your notebook. Highlight the exercises that affect you most, repeating these as often as you'd like, reaping additional benefits each time.

Samples are shown for color coding information in your notebook, as an exercise may remind you of a discovery from a former exercise that you want to revisit. Use my color coding, or feel free to create a coding system of your own that eases your search when you want to locate an exercise later.

I've titled the exercises and listed them in the appendix in the back of the book. If you forget to code an exercise you can locate it through the appendix. I've also expanded the index so you can search by key words. Throughout the book, I include examples of the results of exercises from other caregivers.

DO EXERCISES ALONE OR IN GROUPS?

You can move through the exercises alone, with a counselor, with another caregiver, or with a group of caregivers. Whether a group is led by a professional or not, as caregivers share their insights, everyone benefits. If you decide to read through the book and apply what you've learned with other caregivers, but without a leader, follow these basic self-help group guidelines.

- Limit speaking to one person at a time.
- Avoid giving advice.
- Use "I" statements.
- As others comment, accept what you like and disregard the rest, and encourage others to do the same.
- Don't comment on each other's comments.
- Close the meeting with well-wishes for each other and for all caregivers in the world.
- Then, informally share ideas and observations among members.

When group members start cross-talking or giving advice, more assertive members dominate the group, and more passive members begin to drift away, causing leaderless groups to fall apart. Most people want to help, and offer advice believing they know what they'd do in the same situation. Until they're in the same situation, however, they may give advice that isn't helpful. Unsolicited advice often forces members to defend or try strategies that aren't applicable to their situation. If one person at a time speaks, without cross-talk or advice, each sharing their own experiences by using "I" statements, your group will flourish, and all will benefit. Everyone will be able to take what fits, and leave the rest for a later time or not at all.

RURAL CAREGIVERS

If you're in a rural area, without access to a lot of other caregivers, you can connect with others on the Internet or the phone, taking turns sharing stories, struggles, lessons learned, and services discovered. Weave Maya's Model through your life, your personality, your struggles, and your situation.

MEN CAREGIVERS, WOMEN CAREGIVERS

Although the number of men in the role of caregiving is on the rise, more caregivers are women. Therefore, I refer to the caregiver as "she" and "her." I hope the men who read this will not feel slighted. I've included stories from men caregivers. Studies show that men and women often have different needs related to social support. But, because this model can be woven through each person's needs, it's equally useful for men as women.

This book introduces to you Maya's Model, useful for all caregivers, male and female, old and young, parents, partners, or children, those who prefer fewer people, as well as those who like lots of people, those who are private and those who are very open. Maya's Model is for everyone whose social support network isn't currently providing the support needed.

FONTS AND FORMATS

The following typographical styles have been used to make using this book easier:

- Narrative—The main text and narrative of the book are done in this font, Times.
- Exercises—All the exercises are done in this font, Arial.
- *Caregiver's Stories—All the caregiver's stories are done in this font, Times Italics.*
- **Headings—All the headings are in this font, Times Bold.**
- Examples of Mind Maps/Legends—You'll find samples of handwritten Mind Maps, as a few examples of the endless ways that others' Mind Maps will be different from yours.

Maya's Story

EACH CAREGIVER HAS A PERSONAL STORY TO TELL. HERE'S MINE.

It was a gorgeous day at Eagle Creek Resort and Conference Center in downstate Illinois. I'd finished my presentation on "Empowering Women." My husband, Eddie, and I were eating in the restaurant overlooking the forest and lake. We were looking forward to three days of soaking up the sun and hiking the trails. He went back to the buffet table for more food, while I stared out the window, happily absorbed in the brilliant blue sky and beautiful lush greens surrounding the sparkling lake.

"Excuse me, ma'am," said the hostess. "Your husband seems to have had a seizure." The rest is a blur. Through my shock and anxiety I heard snatches of questions and comments. Does he take medicine? Something about the house doctor. Something about an ambulance.

Our lives would never be the same.

The next six months were a whirlwind. We charged through doctor's offices, hospitals, and Internet searches looking for answers, chasing down yet another approach. Hopes dashed, frustration mounting to a screaming roar, we ran out of theories, we ran out of sick and vacation days, we ran out of money, we ran out of hope, we ran out of energy, and still no conclusions. I thought nothing could be worse than the anguish of not knowing, until I heard the doctor's words, "It's an inoperable tumor. He has about six months to live."

It can't be true. This can't be happening to us. He's only 50 years old. I vacillated between disbelief and ugly reality. No matter what life dished out to us, Eddie and I ended each day cuddling and chatting in the comfort of each other's arms, certain our love could conquer all.

As the tumor grew, Eddie's seizures and periods of confusion increased in duration and intensity, leaving disasters in their wake.

The Frog

Drop a frog in hot water and he will jump out and scurry away. But, place the frog in lukewarm water and slowly turn up the heat, and you can boil him to death without fuss or fanfare. The incremental changes in temperature go unnoticed until too late.

Walk with me through my story of near-destruction, the mistakes I made, and the lessons I learned that evolved into the model I present you, Caregiver, unsung hero that you are.

One day he bought and changed a bunch of locks and had several sets of keys made. He didn't color code the new keys, and immediately lost them amid thousands of keys in boxes in the basement. He often forgot where he put the car. It was towed several times in a few weeks. All too often he'd get lost and call me at work to guide him home.

Over the next year we staggered through treatments, tests, surgery, emergency rooms, each time begging life to give us just a few more months. Laser surgery slowed down the growth of the tumor, giving us more time but prolonging his suffering.

Like a team in a three-legged race, we hobbled along, bobbing and weaving, often in different directions. It was like having a 220-pound two-year-old, occasionally still a grownup. The adult was showing up less often, the child more frequently. All of the rituals and routines I tried to put in place to keep him safe were failing. My life was becoming full-time damage control. The problems were mounting as rapidly as my energy was fading.

One day, he fell and was wedged between the wall and the dresser, crying out in pain. I pushed, shoved, and heaved with all my might, unable to budge him or the humongous dresser. Screaming for a neighbor's help, it took us—Eddie, the neighbor, and me—hours to free him and calm him down.

Another time I came home at the end of the day, opened the door, and found him walking on broken glass, a dazed look in his eyes. Just as I started guiding him to safety, he had a seizure. He fell on top of me, crushing both of us onto the glass. My winter coat, though ruined, had cushioned us both from much worse.

Occasionally he talked about his impending death. Mostly he was in denial, certain a solution was just around the corner. Other times we'd burst into tears and cry in each other's arms—forsaken and traumatized, each by our respective heartache of the same experience.

Nighttime was vicious. I fell asleep from exhaustion, but didn't sleep well, one ear always open for Eddie's call. He'd fall down, and I'd spend half the night trying to lift him back into bed or calm his emotional storms. Sleep deprivation was taking its toll on me. The occasional solid night's sleep no longer replenished me.

I'd break into tears at work. My boss, Melanie Whitter, a kind, compassionate, and supportive woman, requested that personnel put me on seven-day-work-week status, allowing me to put in my 40 hours whenever I could, instead of following the usual start and stop times. What a precious gift. I'd go into the office at odd hours, early mornings, Saturday or Sunday, whenever I could find respite for Eddie.

Seeing the wreck that I was, friends and coworkers would say, "You've got to take better care of yourself."

I wanted to scream, "Tell me how!"

At lunch one day a friend of ours, Dr. Brian Rooney, asked, "Is anyone helping you?" I burst into tears. My "no" was barely audible through my sobbing.

He listened patiently, then told me, "Studies show that caregivers become ill from the stress." He shared research from his dissertation on the benefits of something he called a *social support network*, something he could clearly see that I lacked.

His words echoed back over the next few days. Eddie had already lived a year and a half longer than expected. I began to see that, in many ways, I was deteriorating faster than he was. His brain tumor and impending death were the focus. My colds, flu, and backaches seemed petty by comparison. Little did I know my symptoms were signaling a ticking time bomb in me.

Ceaseless worry drained me. I was exhausted from doctors' appointments, schedule changes, and instant rallying when Eddie had a seizure or period of confusion, all of which were happening more frequently. Before Eddie's illness, I loved meeting new people. I was friendly and talkative. But after almost a year of caregiving, even familiar faces evoked anxiety. I dreaded the phone, fearing demands and unsolicited advice from those unwilling to do anything but meddle. I was irritable and impatient all the time.

I'd been in the habit of starting each day with prayer and meditation. Since Eddie's illness, I'd wake up late, dash out the door, often trying to pray and meditate on the L train going to work. During lunch hour, I'd often go a church nearby, searching to understand God's will in the midst of it all. Sometimes I'd rage at God, sometimes I'd feel peace, more often a sense of wearying emptiness, that I'd been forsaken.

One evening I left my office in downtown Chicago, trudging down the five blocks to the bus, a walk I once enjoyed. On that day I was weary and short of breath, my legs weak and shaky, my eyes searching for the next building, pole, or fire plug I could grab, if necessary. The journey was long and strenuous. I inched wearily toward the L train, fearful I'd collapse.

I arrived home, dragged myself up the stairs to face more "important" crises. A scheduling screw-up with caregivers had left Eddie alone and hysterical. I calmed him, fed him, gave him his medicine, gave him a sponge bath, put in a load of laundry, and crashed into bed.

That fitful night I dreamed I was homeless, hauling all of my worldly possessions on my back, wandering through downtown Chicago searching for a place to rest. Passersby loaded more stuff on my back, saying, "Here, carry this for me." Or, "Here, this is yours." Or, "I'm tired of carrying this," thrusting their burdens onto my breaking back.

Trying to escape the crowds, I staggered down the stairs into a dark, dank subway, gasping for air, my shaky legs weakening more every second. I struggled not to topple over, as people passing on the stairs heaped more onto my breaking back.

Suddenly I was in a deserted section of the subway, terrified, uncertain which direction would lead to safety, too weak to climb back up the stairs, too scared to go forward into the unknown. My body hurt; my arms, my back, my shoulders strained under the weight of the load. I crept along the dark and menacing subway tunnel trembling, barely able to stay afoot. My rubbery legs caved in. I toppled over and died.

I woke up gasping for life and crying. I jumped out of bed and poured every detail I could recall into my journal. I started to see my caregiving burdens as weight, growing heavier as I grew weaker. Some of the burdens were not mine to carry, but I carried them just the same. Struggling alone with broken promises, medication errors, hospital bills, and insurance company mistakes, if I were to survive, I'd have to start unloading, and fast. Between the lack of sleep and lack of support, I was running on empty, weakening and falling further behind every day.

Eventually my childlike faith in people had given way to fear, cynicism, and bitterness. I resented those who were unkind to us, but I felt guilty for feeling that way. Embarrassed about how bad I looked, felt, and acted, I was withdrawing from everyone, even supportive and loving friends.

Picking up Eddie when he fell was beyond my physical capabilities, taking hours, yet this was something I forced myself to do as he was falling more often. I'd shove him toward the bed, prop blankets and pillows under him. He'd use his one good arm, I'd heave ho and shove more props under him. Eventually, through exhaustive efforts by the two of us, we'd get him back in bed. I dreaded nights, fearful of such crises. I dreaded mornings because I was exhausted, but had to go to work.

One night during a seizure, he fell and cut his head open pretty bad, and I had to call an ambulance. Two paramedics walked in, took one look at the size of Eddie and requested a third guy. I was stunned, suddenly realizing that what I'd been doing for months wasn't reasonable. Is it normal to have so little regard for myself that all 5'4", 140 pounds of me kept trying to lift his 6'1", 220-pound body back into bed? What was wrong with me?

During that year and a half, his left arm became completely paralyzed, his left leg growing progressively weaker. He had to go into a nursing home. That was obvious, yet I hated myself for thinking that, knowing he'd feel abandoned and betrayed.

Loving, supportive friends and neighbors offered to help. If only I'd known how to make better use of their offers. I thought that a support network was something that one simply *had*, certainly nothing to be questioned or worked on systematically. Certain people were helpful. Others were not.

My dream forced me to face my own failing health. Brian Rooney's compassion and understanding brought insightful relief. I'd been running on empty for a long time and my body was rebelling. Brian opened up a new world with the idea that I could create the support that I needed. His words rattled around in my head, and over the following months began to bear fruit.

I started using Mind Mapping™ (discussed in Chapter 2), a technique I'd learned years before and used for managing complex multiple projects at work. Why, I wondered, hadn't I thought of Mind Mapping before? I played around with ideas for color coding, and how to use Mind Mapping to manage the avalanche of demands.

I identified toxic feelings of guilt and unworthiness from my childhood, played out through my compulsive need to put others first. In time I faced the harsh reality that Eddie needed a nursing home. Our friends came to the rescue again. Mike and Roger stayed with Eddie, while Lynne and I traipsed through dirty, depressing, cold, unfriendly nursing homes. Some homes we looked at were filled with residents who looked terrified and reeked of urine. We searched until we found a home that was cheerful and clean, had good food, flexible visiting hours, and—most important of all—where the interactions between staff and residents appeared warm and friendly. Everything inside of me railed against placing him, but I struggled through the financial and medical arrangements, and set the date for his admission. Hard as that was, it was the easy part.

The next day, when he was admitted, was devastating. My friends described me as shell-shocked. I'd been losing him to the brain cancer a little at a time. But now I was abandoning him, my partner, my buddy. For days afterward I couldn't function. Confused and disoriented, missing Eddie terribly, I spent every free minute at the nursing home. I was stunned and frustrated at how much I had to advocate for him, monitor his care, call for and pressure staff to respond to his needs. The staff was kind, but scanty, so crises preempted or delayed low-priority requests. But, many of those so-called "low priority" requests offered comfort for the anguish of being taken from his home.

Back at home I pushed myself through tons of neglected tasks. With the help of friends I sold our house and moved into a condo. I joined a caregivers' support group, and became more self-protective. I found the courage to stand up to some health care professionals, and I pushed some troublesome people out of my life.

My friends held my life together. I burned up the phone wires constantly, pouring my heartache out to my two closest friends, Lynne and Deann. I had lunch with Brian whenever our schedules jibed, and I bent his ear. My girlfriend Dawn, a massage therapist, had been offering me free massages for months, but there simply wasn't time. After Eddie went into the nursing home I started going to Dawn's every Sunday morning for a massage, relishing her motherly tenderness. Her unconditional acceptance and nurturing unleashed my pent-up tears and intense grief.

Denial protected Eddie from the harsh reality, but it also prevented him from accepting the supportive services of hospice. The day he finally signed the hospice papers, I climbed in his bed at the nursing home. We cuddled, cried, and talked for hours. I felt a little less alone, and tremendous relief, knowing I could let go some. Hospice would partner with me in advocating for Eddie's comfort and safety.

Clinging to each other that day, Eddie cried and said, "I'll be going to the white light soon, but I don't want to go without you." In his rare lucid moments, we still cuddled, chatted, giggled, and processed life. But my buddy was slipping away faster every day.

Despite my newfound awareness, my partners in hospice, and valiant efforts to take better care of myself, I was too late. I collapsed with pneumonia a month before Eddie died. I was too weak to get out of bed to visit him. He deteriorated rapidly. I hated my body for failing me so close to the finish line. Although not very rational, those were my feelings nonetheless.

Later, Sharon McCarthy, the hospice social worker helped me see that my collapsing had two silver linings. She said Eddie was having a hard time dying and letting go of me. In my absence, dying was easier for him. And, for me—while bed-ridden, I started pouring my feelings out on paper, a catharsis of my grief and bitterness, that would no longer be denied.

One day, lying in bed writing in my journal, the TV playing in the background, I stumbled onto an interview with researchers Drs. Janice and Ronald Glaser on the negative impact of caregiving on the immune system. The combination of Brian's dissertation about the protective factors of a *Social Support Network* and the TV interview about the Glasers' research shifted the focus of my journaling. The bitterness began to lift, and gave way to the heart of this book.

Sometimes I'd write furiously, finding relief in writing. Other times I'd back away from the painful reminders. Between grieving, processing the horrors of caregiving, and my health, it was an emotional roller coaster ride for a while. Slowly I returned to my life and career in the addictions field, with this book nipping at my heels. Sometimes I'd sit in front of the computer and stare, unable to write. I'd ignore the book for months at a time. Then begin writing furiously again, as if compelled by some force outside myself.

It took me more than three years after Eddie's death to regain the health, energy, and zest for life I had before his illness. *If Only I'd Had This Caregiving Book*, perhaps my suffering would have been less severe. But if my experience, shared through this model, eases your pain, then it won't have been in vain. It's my *Never Again* book. *Never again for me! Never again for you.* It is my gift to you, Caregiver, unsung hero that you are, to help you survive caregiving.

The Key to Your Survival: Maya's Model

It takes a team of doctors, three shifts of registered nurses, three shifts of nurse's aides, a laundry department, a janitorial department, a delivery department, a lab, and a pharmacy department to do the same things a caregiver is expected to accomplish when the patient is discharged.
—*Billie Jackson*, The Caregivers' Roller Coaster

ARE YOU A TICKING TIME BOMB?

Under the best of circumstances, caregiving is tough: endless physical demands, sleepless nights, the mental stress of worrying, juggling all the pieces, the heartache of watching your loved one suffer. Under the mounting pressure it's no wonder caregivers themselves become ill.

Studies show that caregivers have weaker immune systems than a group with similar characteristics who aren't caregivers. The immune system weakness may show up as perpetual colds, flu bugs, aches, or pains. Or worse yet, under the lash of caregiving, genetic weaknesses such as diabetes, cancer, or heart disease may be given the opportunity to flourish.

BUT THERE'S HOPE!

The research of John B. Jemmott, Ph.D., and Kim K. Magliore, Ph.D., showed that college students with a "satisfying" social support network (SSN) produced more antibodies than students who expressed dissatisfaction with their SSNs. And antibodies are important because they give the body its ability to fight off encroaching illness or disease.

If you're lucky enough to have scads of money, help, and loving support to share your caregiving burdens, you could probably fare pretty well. But if you're like most caregivers, you don't have enough support, or not the right kind at the right time. A study sponsored by the National Alliance for Caregivers and the American Association of Retired Persons found that one in five caregivers say their relatives are not doing their share, and 31 percent say no one else helps or they get some help from a non-relative.

If you're among those caregivers receiving little or no help, it's time to take a stand. Those activities you've graciously given up aren't frivolous at all, they're medicine for your immune system, essential to your survival. The goal is to fit those pleasurable activities back into your life *and* manage caregiving by creating an effective social support network (SSN). All this is possible by applying Maya's Model.

In this chapter you'll be given an opportunity to sample Maya's Model, which has four components: You, Your To-Do List, and Your Social Support Network, and Mind Mapping. In the following chapters you'll delve deeper to understand and apply each component of the model, to ease the stress and strengthen the support to thrive and survive caregiving.

YOU DESERVE THE BEST!

Because you selflessly give your life to the care of your loved one, I believe that you deserve all the needed help, money, resources, and physical and emotional support, and I believe that no one should be allowed to make caregiving harder for you. But, what's more important is that *you believe*. The following is a list of my beliefs that caregivers deserve the best of everything, including love, respect, and plenty of help. As you review these 10 statements, what comes to mind? Take out your notebook and journal about your feelings and reactions to these beliefs. Do you agree? Do you disagree?

EXERCISE: You Deserve the Best!

I believe you deserve everything in the following statements. But, do you agree? As you review these, notice how you feel, and what you think, and if you agree or disagree.

1. I believe that as primary caregiver, dedicating time and other resources to the care of your loved one, orchestrating and coordinating all aspects of your lives, that you are the one person who understands what works, what doesn't, and why.
    AGREE   DISAGREE

2. I believe you are worthy and deserving of a life of your own, including the people, places, things, and activities you enjoy.
    AGREE   DISAGREE

3. I believe you deserve all the money you need, all the help you need, and all the support you need.
    AGREE   DISAGREE

4. I believe you have a right to have and express all of your emotions (sadness, anger, joy, fear) whether or not others understand or agree.
    AGREE   DISAGREE

5. I believe you have a unique set of skills, abilities, likes, dislikes, and capabilities, with an inner wisdom about the ideal way to resolve the issues in your life, because you alone understand the needs and limitations of your situation.
    AGREE   DISAGREE

6. I believe you have a right to object when others try to tell you how to think, act, or feel, and that no one else has a right to judge you or insist that you do things their way.
    AGREE   DISAGREE

7. I believe that you'll benefit most from those who accept and value you exactly as you are.
    AGREE   DISAGREE

8. I believe you should be able to honor the wishes of your loved one as you and your loved one agree, without having to justify or explain your decisions to others, especially those who don't live with your situation on a daily basis.

    AGREE　　　　DISAGREE

9. I believe you have a right to exclude from your life anyone who meddles, gossips, judges, interferes, or in any other way makes caregiving more difficult for you.

    AGREE　　　　DISAGREE

10. I believe you are entitled to elicit help from others, and delegate to those you choose, any tasks that they and you agree on, without having to justify those decisions to others.

    AGREE　　　　DISAGREE

11. I believe you have a right to have friends and allies to advocate/intervene for you with people who increase the stress of your caregiving burdens.

    AGREE　　　　DISAGREE

ARE YOU ENTITLED?

As someone who has been through the tough role of caregiver, I sincerely believe that you are entitled to everything stated above. But do you believe that? In the following exercise, you are being asked to review each of the statements and your notes, and to rate your reactions. Believing you are entitled and enforcing these rights can reduce your stress. Feeling undeserving or conflicted can increase your stress.

Hopefully, you already agree, and express appreciation to those who treat you with the respect embodied in these statements, and you're able to let others know about the negative impact on you and your situation when they don't. If you have difficulty feeling entitled to or enforcing these rights, press on. Maya's Model is designed to help you strengthen your own belief in these rights.

EXERCISE: Rate Your Responses to Caregiver's Rights

- Review each of the caregiver's rights.
- What reactions did you have to each of the caregiver's rights?
- Rate yourself according to the category you see yourself in.

    A.　　I agree with this right.

    ◊　　I honor this right.

    ◊　　I let others know I appreciate it when they respect it.

    ◊　　I let others know when they violate this right.

    B.　　Mostly I agree.

    ◊　　I don't agree entirely (journal about your thoughts and feelings, the ways you agree and/or disagree).

    ◊　　Or I agree, but have difficulty letting others know how I feel when they don't honor this right (journal about why you find it difficult to let others know how you feel).

    C.　　I don't agree.

    ◊　　Or, I'm struggling with conflicting beliefs.

    ◊　　Or, I have underlying beliefs (such as unworthiness or powerlessness) that need to be changed before I could completely believe in this right.

Take out your journal and write your thoughts and feelings about the rights you rated as B, or C. Describe why it's difficult for you to feel entitled to that right and any strategies you might employ to help you believe you are entitled to that right.

A   If your ratings are mostly A's, that's great! You have enough self protectiveness that you probably balance your needs with the needs of your loved one, and you deal effectively with people who try to violate your rights.

B   If you have a lot of B's, you may already implement many of the strategies in this book. But, through the exercises in the book you can strengthen your self-protectiveness, and your right to the support you need and turn those B's into A's.

C   If you have C's, explore the negative impact of not believing you have that right, by journaling about your thoughts and feelings. Why don't you feel entitled? Explore the ways your life would be different or better if you did believe in that right. Do you know when or how in your past the limiting belief was formed?

MAYA'S MODEL

The three components of the model are You, Your To-Do List, and Your Social Support Network. See Figure 1. As you assess and strengthen each component using Mind Mapping, you'll be surprised and delighted as creative solutions emerge.

Maya's Model also uses Mind Mapping, (see figure 1) a viewing lens that elicits insights and solutions from your creative self, helping you identify needs and resources, and implement the ideal solutions for you and your situation.

YOU—Your unique gifts, abilities, traits, skills, talents, likes, and dislikes are important to know in order to honor your rights and secure the kind of "Support" you need.

YOUR TO-DO LIST—You'll create Mind Maps to know at a glance what needs to be done, who has volunteered for which chores, and tasks still needing volunteers.

YOUR SSN—Your SSN is made up of all the people, resources, and potential resources in your SSN. The exercises will help you list the people, identify their particular skills, and link those to the tasks on your list.

Now that you have an overview of Maya's Model, let's sample Mind Mapping, a creative method to extract solutions and enhance harmony between you, your To-Do List, and your SSN.

First we'll look at each component separately, then collectively. The exercises will help you strengthen your social support network, so it will adjust and adapt to the ever-changing demands of caregiving.

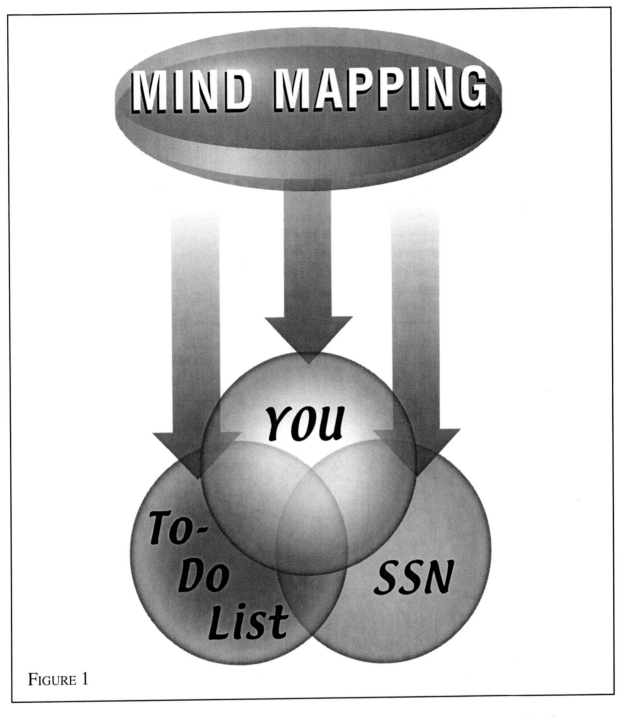

FIGURE 1

The goal of Maya's Model is to increase your support, self protectiveness, and self caring so you can weather the storms of caregiving. There are three components, as shown in figure 1:

- You—Maya's Model helps you identify your needs, wants, strengths, and weaknesses. They are a unique combination that is YOU, the caregiver.
- Your To-Do List— Using Mind Mapping to get a handle on your To-Do List, also unique to you, your situation, your family, and the loved one you care for.
- Your Social Support Network (SSN)—Your SSN will be also be unique to you, made up of your friends, family, coworkers, and acquaintances from church, school, and the community, including the services that are available or lacking in your community.

MIND MAPPING

Mind Mapping is an easy, fun method for creatively tapping the answers within. No two caregivers have the same personalities, same needs, same problems, or the same resources. Mind Mapping will help you clarify the perfect solutions for *you* and *your* situation. Let's sample Mind Mapping.

EXERCISE: Mind Map the Wonders of You

- On a clean page in your notebook write your name in the center with a circle around it (see figure 2).
- Draw spokes out from the center, attaching words that describe your qualities, gifts, talents, skills, abilities, likes, and interests (see figure 2).
- Add spokes, listing and circling words until you run out of descriptions of you (see figure 2).
- Next, think about at least three people who love and value you.
- Add positive things they would say (see figure 3).

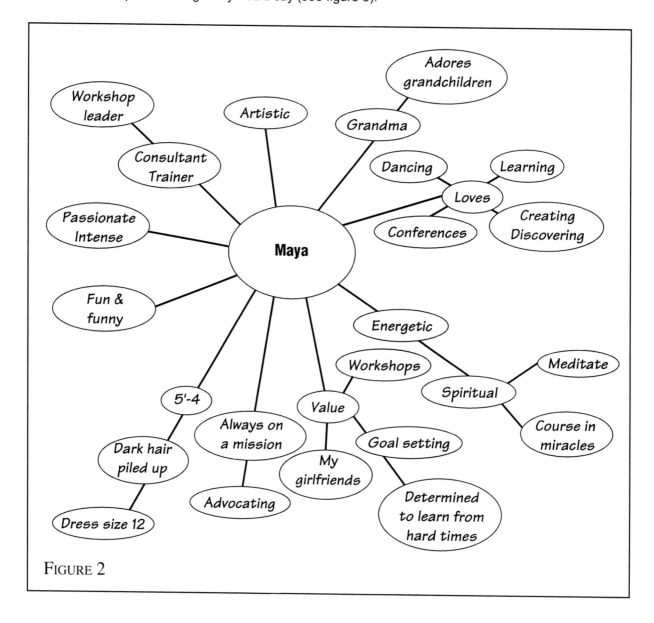

FIGURE 2

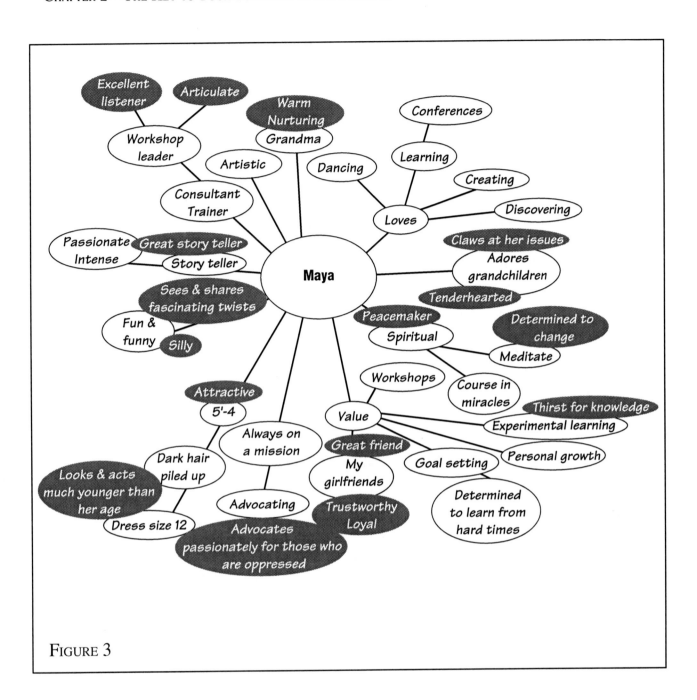

FIGURE 3

Now you've created your first Mind Map. There is no one else quite like you. No one else in the world has your unique combination of traits, gifts, skills, and qualities. Keep this *Mind Map of the Wonders of You*. In the next chapter you'll take Mind Mapping to the next level, learning more about this easy yet profound method for tapping your own creative solutions.

WHAT IS A SOCIAL SUPPORT NETWORK?

A social support network is a complex web of people, needs, and interactions. How you describe, assess, and improve your own network will be unique to you and your situation, rather than upon some "official" notion of what an SSN "ought" to be. Social Support Networks (SSNs) that are considered *effective and satisfying* consist of relationships that include helpful elements such as: support in managing emotional pain, sharing tasks, providing supplies such as money, meals, materials, tools, skills, and/or guidance to help you manage particular situations.

EXERCISE: Is Your Current SSN Helpful?

Rate each of these four types of support on a scale of 1-5, five being the ideal amount of support.

Little or None	/	Not nearly enough	/	Some/Need more	/	Almost	/	Enough Support
1		2		3		4		5

- Emotional support
- Help with tasks
- Needed supplies (money, equipment)
- Guidance

ARE YOU SATISFIED WITH YOUR SSN?

Social Support Networks (SSNs) that are effective, sustaining, and satisfying are **reciprocal** between you and the people in your network. Because the relationships are reciprocal, everyone in the network gladly shares resources, and feels free to ask for help when its needed. This sharing and asking for help makes it easy for everyone in the SSN to be there for one another.

If we're exceptionally lucky, everyone we love will love everyone else we love. All of our relationships will be reciprocal, fulfilling, rising with us to meet any challenge. For most of us reality is different. Our network is a mixture of people, ranging from loving and supportive to those whose presence adds tension.

Take out a notebook and pen, and write the name of the exercise and the page number from this book. Then begin writing down the thoughts, feelings, examples, and anything that comes up as you proceed through this exercise. Writing down your thoughts, feelings and reactions to all the exercises is a free form of "journaling," that studies show is helpful in problem solving.

EXERCISE: Are You Satisfied with Your Social Support Network?

Journal/write about your responses to the following questions.

- Are you satisfied with the number of people in your SSN?
- Are you satisfied with the kind of support they provide?
- What would be helpful to improve the support you get from the people in your network?

Review your answers (above) and compare them with responses from other caregivers (below) and the suggested solutions.

OTHER CAREGIVERS

Are you satisfied with the number of people in your SSN?

No! There are too many people demanding too much from me.

Solutions:

- *I'll find out once and for all who sincerely wants to help.*
- *I'll tell my sister I can't be there for her now and ask for her help.*
- *I'll have my older kids help each other more and depend on me less.*

No! There are not enough people to help with the increasing demands.

Solutions:

- *I'll reach out to more people, beginning with people I've helped in the past.*
- *I'll contact social service agencies in the area to see what's available and affordable.*
- *I'll contact organizations such as NFCA (National Family Caregivers Association), American Cancer Society, Area Agencies on Aging, Alzheimer's.*

Are you satisfied with the kind of support they provide?

No! Some people offer help, but don't come through. I'm not sure if they're sincere.

Solutions:

- *I'll find out once and for all who sincerely wants to help.*
- *I'll find out what each potential helper would be most comfortable doing.*

No! Some people seem genuinely concerned, but their advice shows they don't really understand my situation.

Solutions:

- *I'll ask for help with specific tasks, and see if they come through.*
- *I'll be honest and tell them I don't find unsolicited advice useful.*

If other thoughts, feelings, or solutions occur to you as you read responses from other caregivers, feel free to journal or write about it. Record the name of each exercise and the page number from this book, so you can find it later.

WHAT DOES SUPPORT MEAN TO YOU?

Support means different things to different people. At its best, a SSN will provide you with the security of knowing that whatever comes up, the people in your SSN will rise with you to meet it, and that your SSN will adapt to the ever-changing conditions of caregiving. Grab a pen and let's begin. Write down the name of the exercise and the page number from this book.

EXERCISE: Supportive People in Your Life?

List some supportive people in your life in each of the following categories:

- Current
- Past

One common but troublesome aspect of human nature is we assume that other people want what we want and need what we need. To illustrate how one's cup of tea may be another's cup of poison, here are a few possible examples of support.

- Offers of help
- Advice
- Listening
- Information
- Guidance
- Money
- Supplies
- Physical presence
- Taking over some tasks
- Telling others about your situation
- Not telling others about your situation without your permission
- Being asked questions (i.e., expressing interest, or opening dialogue)
- Not being asked questions (because it feels intrusive)

EXERCISE: What Do You Consider "Supportive?"

- Review the above list.
- Circle the types of support most helpful to you.
- Cross out the least helpful.
- Add other things you consider helpful and supportive.

There are no wrong answers. It's all personal preference. What one person considers support, another finds stressful. Maya's Model is about understanding, honoring, and creating the type of support that you need.

YOUR TO-DO LIST

In the following exercise you'll create a Mind Map of your To-Do List, all the tasks, large and small, you have to do, including your needs and the needs of your loved ones. Creating a Mind Map will help you organize what has to be done.

EXERCISE: A Mind Map of Your "To-Do List"

- Take a piece of paper and write "To-Do List" in the center and circle it (see figure 4).
- Then draw spokes from that center and begin jotting down everything you can think of that's on your current to-do list.
- Next, take two different colored pens or pencils, and code the items as either (see figure 4)
  - ◊ Light   Easy for you to do
  - ◊ Heavy Difficult for you to do

Bill: Everybody said it's easy to give shots, you'll get used to it, but I never did. I was in a panic all the hours leading up to her shot. I'd have nightmares about hitting a wrong spot and killing her. Weeks later I heard Maya say, if there's something you don't want to do, shift it ASAP. A nurse in the neighborhood offered to come over and give my wife her heparin shots. Now I sleep like a baby.

Jenny: My husband took care of our finances until the accident. I tried but found it unnerving. Friends insisted I could master a simple bookkeeping course, but it made me more anxious. My daughter came over to help with housework. I asked if she'd do the bookkeeping instead, and I'd do the housework. What a burden lifted that day.

Alice: My two sisters and I share caregiving for our mother who is dying of leukemia. I do a lot, always have, but I've never had any children, and changing diapers gags me. I felt like I was being unreasonable. Finally my sister and I talked. I discovered tasks she dreads a lot more than diapering, like dealing with social service agencies. She shifted those things to me. Now we're both happy.

Shift those "heavy" items quickly. If you rated an item as "heavy" because it's very emotional, share it with someone you trust who's a good listener and/or write about it. Talking and writing can ease emotional pain, paving the way to insights. Ask a supportive ally to intervene and deal with a difficult person for you. Accept offers of help. Delegate what you can, as fast as you can, to those with the right skills. As you lighten the load by shifting or sharing, the remaining items won't feel so crushing.

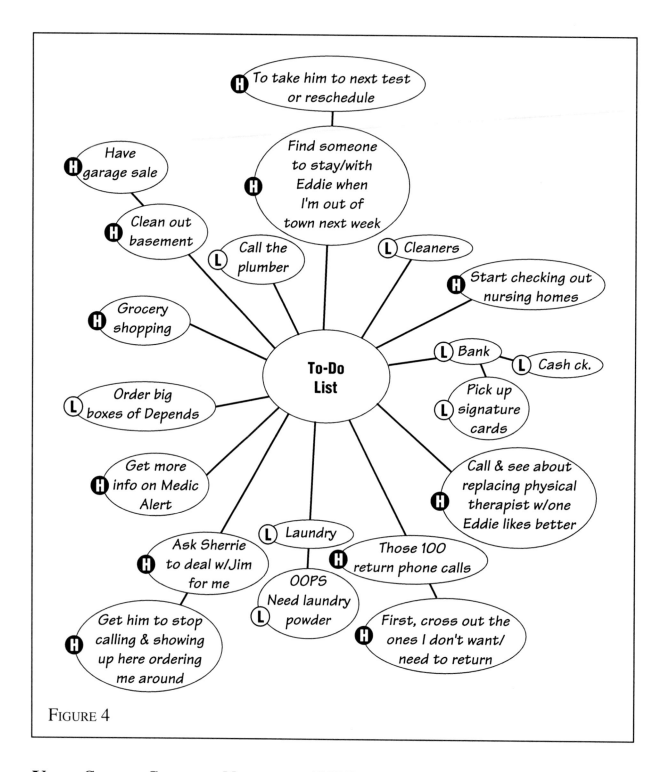

FIGURE 4

YOUR SOCIAL SUPPORT NETWORK (SSN) AND YOUR TO-DO LIST

Most social networks evolve through the years around our life patterns, likes, and dislikes. They may include close friends, family members, and friends of our family members. They can also include acquaintances, coworkers, colleagues, neighbors, and members of organizations to which we or our family members belong, such as volunteer groups, self-help groups, churches or other spiritual organizations, fraternities and sororities, and civic organizations like the Chamber of Commerce. What other categories of people are in your Social Support Network?

EXERCISE: Mind Mapping Your SSN

- Write "My SSN" in the center of a page, and circle it.
- Draw spokes from the center and write names of people you could turn to for help.
- Take out your To-Do List Mind Map and place it side by side with this Mind Map.
- Study the two maps.
- Look for links between people and tasks.
- When you see a link, ask the person for help.
- Or, journal about what stops you from asking certain people for help.

Under normal conditions your SSN might include too many people or not enough, a mixture of fun times and occasional disappointments, but no major problems. When life is "normal," you easily overlook annoying traits of some people. But, under the lash of caregiving perhaps your patience gives out. Be kind to yourself, especially now, during the stress of caregiving. Instead of berating yourself, limit your contact with stressful people when possible.

Geri: When my mom was dying I thought I didn't have enough people in my SSN. Afraid others would think I was a complainer, I didn't share how bad things were. I applied Maya's model. With my to-do list in hand, when someone offered help, I'd rattle off my list. I was amazed at how quickly people offered help. Some took over some tasks entirely, others recruited teams to provide me with respite. An older lady from Mom's church group volunteered to visit and bring Mom her favorite sugar-free desserts once a week.

EXERCISE: What Do I Like/Dislike Doing?

Review each item on your to-do list, and ask yourself the following questions:

- Is this something I prefer to do?
- Is this something I'd prefer NOT to do?
- Could this item be shifted to someone else?
- Does it require me and only me?
- Is it a one-time task?

Here are a few answers to the question in the preceding exercise from other caregivers.

Beth: I discovered that I'm not the only who could sort through medical bills or fold laundry.

Wanda: A well-timed visitor for him would free me up to go to the hairdresser, dentist, or take some desperately needed leisure time.

Tom: I wished I had someone to cook once in awhile so my wife and I could have some time together in the evening. A friend was happy to help. Sometimes she cooked at our house. Sometimes she brought over a dish already cooked.

Vicky: I wasn't strong enough to bathe my husband. Two of his friends and I bathed him together. We had fun, got silly. After that his friends came back a couple times a week and bathed him without me. I gave him sponge baths in-between. They enjoyed the time together, and I was free to do other chores.

Shift a Task Every Day

Start shifting tasks now! And keep shifting tasks every day. Think of tasks, issues, and problems in terms of weight. Some things that only take a few minutes may be draining physically or emotionally. For example, Kathy asked her minister to sit with her during a dreaded discussion with her adult children about their father's condition and deterioration, a task she been putting off for weeks. The session went well, and afterward Kathy said she felt a "weight lifted."

Other things on your list might be time-consuming, but not stressful. For example, Beth prefers doing her own laundry, but it's time-consuming. She gave laundry a higher weight because of the time it takes. Dealing with health care professionals was higher weight, though it took less time, because she felt intimidated by "experts."

So, grab your pen and notebook, and do the following exercise to find out how heavy your tasks are.

EXERCISE: "Heavy/Pressing Items" on Your To-Do List

- Put an (H) next to the items you consider heavy or pressing.
  Put an (L) next to the ones that you consider light, less of a burden, or less urgent.

  ◊ Who in your network has offered the needed help?

    Reach out to them.

  ◊ Who has the needed skills?

    Reach out and ask for their help.

  ◊ Can you shift something today?

    If so, put your pen down and go ask for help.

  ◊ Talk some of these over with others.

    Who do you feel comfortable talking to?

  ◊ Remember the heavier items on your to-do list, and mention those first when someone asks if they can help.

This exercise provided a sample of questions to help you creatively link people with chores, and recognize what goes into shifting chores. What was your reaction? Did you have trouble thinking of people with the required skills? Did you feel uncomfortable about asking? We'll get deeper into linking people and chores, and barriers to shifting tasks, as you move through the exercises in the rest of the chapters.

Have you felt compelled to give up people, places, or activities that once brought you pleasure? These are medicine for your psyche. They strengthen your immune system. As you move through Maya's Model, asking for and securing help, shifting and delegating, you and your loved one will both benefit. You'll have room in your life to resume pleasurable, antibody-producing activities that were squeezed out by caregiving.

CLOSING

In this chapter you've sampled Maya's Model (You, Your To-Do List, and Your SSN, with Mind Mapping), and the power of getting these components working together for you.

The next chapter is all about "support." As humans we need the support of others. And at different times in our lives, such as caregiving, those needs can be very different. So let's proceed to

Developing a Network of Support

WHAT IS SUPPORT?

Like Maggie I had lots of friends who stood by feeling helpless, watching me deteriorate into anxiety, depression, exhaustion, social withdrawal, and mounting health problems of my own. They cared. They were willing to help. But they were not sure how. I was too busy thrashing my way through the crises to see their caring. I desperately needed help, but planning was out of the question. I didn't have time to do the things I needed to do. Of course I didn't have time to plan. Or so I thought.

Near self-destruction I faced it—I wasn't going to survive caregiving unless I created an efficient and effective Social Support Network (SSN). Slowly I began to see the wisdom in the methods for creating a sustaining SSN. It was unique to me. It efficiently blended the needs, limitations and personal preferences of my personality, along with the To-Do List of my loved one and me, and a means of accessing the loving support in our SSN.

Imagine if you had a network that was supportive and helpful, that would be uniquely yours, making caregiving easier. Imagine what that supportive, efficient, effective network of resources would look like, sound like, feel like. For each caregiver, the vision would be as unique as her personality. In this chapter we're going to take you through a series of exercises to help you define a supportive network.

We'll begin by defining "support." The following comments from caregivers are a few examples of what others consider support. Following the caregivers' quotes is an exercise to help you clarify what support has meant to you in the past, and to use those past experiences to become clearer about what support is required now to meet your needs.

Grab your journal/notebook and your pen, and after reading the quotes from other caregivers, consider just one aspect of your Social Support Network: your own definition of "support."

Maggie burst into tears and yelled, "I don't need advice. I need elbow grease! I need sleep!" Her husband was dying. After four months without a full night's sleep, dealing with an avalanche of crises and chores, she was cracking under the pressure. Well-meaning friends stood by feeling helpless wondering what they might do to help Maggie.

Here are examples from other caregivers:

"I've always felt supported by those who share their similar experiences with me. Feeling less alone, I could see my way through an ordeal. Throughout my life, whenever I come upon difficult situations, I am strengthened by those who share their own similar situations"

"When my husband was dying, my sister's presence made me feel safe, secure and confident. In a difficult time, if someone I trust is present I feel supported and can do the next right thing. If no one is present I feel paralyzed, unable to make even the simplest decisions, conflicted about what I'm supposed to do."

"When my husband left me, my neighbor took over chores for me or cared for my children for the first few days while I got though the shock, got my bearings, and figured out what I was supposed to do next. Those first few days were a mixture of shock and confusion. She listened without judgment or advice, and her presence provided a stability to me and my children. That's what my mother used to do when I was a child."

"My best friend knows I don't like to talk when I'm upset. Instead when my mother died, when I got bad news about my health, and when my son was hurt at school, each time she provided transportation, a massage, a meal. These were all quiet assurance that I wasn't alone, making it possible for me to keep going."

"When I lost my job, my brother kept countering my self blame with positive examples of my skills and talents. All my life he's been supportive that way during hard times. When my parents wanted me to go to a different college, and when they didn't like my boyfriend, my brother spoke up for me. I'm quick to doubt myself and back down. He's quick to counter it with solid examples of why my choices should be honored."

"During my divorce, two close girlfriends defended me when others were criticizing me. I was raised in a shaming blaming family. I realized that all my life I've felt most supported by those who defend me."

"After my husband lost his job, friends and family came over with groceries, and offered money, references, and job leads."

"When I've had something scary or challenging in my life, like waiting for test results, I've felt most supported by the people who prayed with me."

"After the fire at our house, I'd wake up frantic during the night needing to talk. I felt most supported by those I could call any time of the day or night. If I didn't call someone I'd be up all night, unable to settle down. If someone could listen, and reassure me, I'd be back to sleep in a matter of minutes."

"My daughter came and sat with me. Never said a word. Just sat with me. She's just like my grandmother, who was my greatest comfort."

"I didn't have to tell her to keep our conversations confidential, she just did. When I can trust someone with my secrets, that makes me feel safe and supported."

So, let's get into the exercise.

EXERCISE: "Support" Then and Now

- List times in the past when you have felt supported. List all the experiences, as far back in time as you can remember.
- Describe the kind of support you received in each experience.
- Write out everything you remember about each experience.
- Who provided you with the needed support?
- What was it about each person that made you feel supported?
- What "support" was provided to you?

Review each event and each person who was supportive. Look for themes to help you understand what "support" meant in the past. From there determine if support looks and feels the same today as it did in the past, and if that same kind of support would ease the stress of your current caregiving situation.

In the book *High Performance Patterns*, author Jerry Fletcher says that our patterns form early, and remain pretty much the same all our lives. Same or similar things are considered supportive even when we compare a situation at age 11 to one at age 25, age 40, or age 60. By determining what made you feel supported at various difficult times in your life, you will be able to seek that same kind of support now, when you need it again.

If being heard is most important to you, seek out good listeners. If advice about quality services you need is most important, locate that information. If respite recharges you, find ways to get those needed breaks. If words of reassurance are what you need, spend more time with those who are reassuring and less time with those who are critical.

Review each event and each person who was supportive that you listed in the exercise. Look for themes to help you understand what support meant to you in the past. From there, determine whether support still looks, feels, and sounds the same for you today.

Here are examples from other caregivers who did this exercise.

Diane: I was amazed to discover that support means the same thing today as it did when I was 12—a nurturing friend, who doesn't sugar-coat reality. And she says, "Tell me what I can do to help." And then she does it! Diane's father has emphysema.

Lynne: Just having someone listen to me. Being heard. That's all. No advice. No analysis. When I share and someone listens, truly listens, solutions emerge, I feel empowered and stronger. There is no greater gift anyone can give me than listening to me. Lynne is caring for a brother with AIDS.

Arlene: After the accident, I was traumatized. I couldn't think. I was immobilized. My best friend Jane jumped in and took over my house and my kids, handled phone calls, scheduled appointments. After two or three days of crying and sleeping, I could think more clearly and gradually took charge of my family again. In each event I revisited, someone I trusted took charge, which got me over the initial hump. Arlene's husband and one child were seriously injured in a car accident.

Joan: When I was 10 years old, my grandmother spotted the bruises all over me, held me close and said, "Those boys shouldn't be mean to you. You're a wonderful little girl." Later, I heard her reprimanding my mother for not protecting me from my older brothers. To this day, when someone stands up for me, I feel loved and valued and better able to handle any situation. Joan's mother is a stroke victim.

ELEMENTS OF AN EFFECTIVE SSN

Studies show that the key elements of an effective and satisfying SSN include companionship, intimacy, confidants, and conflict resolution. In the following exercise, we'll look at each of these four key elements in your SSN, before and since (current or past—if applicable) your caregiving situation began.

When I think of my two best friends—Deann and Lynne—there's great comfort in knowing I can always be myself. I can be happy, sad, scared, angry, or absurd. These friendships have spanned many years, a lifetime of joy and challenges, yet remain intact with unconditional love. These friendships include the following key elements of satisfying social support: companionship, confidants, intimacy, and conflict resolution.

EXERCISE: Satisfied with Your Social Support Network?

As you answer these questions, focusing on companionship, confidentiality, intimacy, and conflict resolution, include the names of people who provide each type of support. Record the name and page number of the exercise in your notebook. Jot down any insights that come up, and/or talk it over with someone.

Companionship

Companionship is sharing with people you enjoy being around, whether it's attending events together, shopping, accompanying each other to appointments, or just hanging out. Who comes to mind as good company when you want to see a movie, a play, a sporting event, go to a party, have someone over for dinner, or other activities? One person? Several different people?

I AM SATISFIED WITH THE COMPANIONSHIP IN MY SSN.

Strongly Agree	Before CG	Since CG
Agree	Before CG	Since CG
Disagree	Before CG	Since CG
Strongly Disagree	Before CG	Since CG
Name(s)		
Comments		

Confidants

Confidants are people you trust, with whom you feel safe to share your secrets. Studies show that having one or more confidants is a key ingredient to a satisfying SSN. As caregiving challenges increase, confidants are essential to your survival. Who comes to mind when you think of someone you safely can share anything with?

I HAVE ONE OR MORE PEOPLE IN MY SSN WHO I TRUST TO
SHARE MY INNERMOST THOUGHTS AND FEELINGS, WHO WILL
NOT JUDGE ME OR DIVULGE MY SECRETS.

Strongly Agree	Before CG	Since CG
Agree	Before CG	Since CG
Disagree	Before CG	Since CG
Strongly Disagree	Before CG	Since CG
Name(s)		
Comments		

Intimacy

Intimacy is an emotional connection and attachment that goes deep, isn't easily broken, and usually includes the above elements of companionship and confidant, as well as reciprocity. Because of the depth of an intimate relationship, when an intimate relationship ends, a person will grieve the loss.

I AM SATISFIED WITH THE DEPTH OF CLOSENESS WITH PEOPLE
I WOULD MISS TERRIBLY IF THEY WERE NO LONGER IN MY LIFE.

Strongly Agree	Before CG	Since CG
Agree	Before CG	Since CG
Disagree	Before CG	Since CG
Strongly Disagree	Before CG	Since CG
Name(s)		
Comments		

Conflict Resolution

True intimacy includes the ability to disagree and a willingness to resolve, negotiate, and compromise to restore harmony. Intimate relationships are not likely to be broken as a result of minor conflict. In healthy as well as unhealthy relationships there is conflict. In healthy relationships, there is also resolution. In unhealthy relationships the conflict goes underground, and may result in retaliation or a resurgence of the same arguments over and over without resolution.

I HAVE RELATIONSHIPS IN WHICH BOTH PARTIES EMPLOY CONFLICT RESOLUTION, SUCH AS NEGOTIATING, COMPROMISING, LISTENING AND RESPECT.

Strongly Agree	Before CG	Since CG
Agree	Before CG	Since CG
Disagree	Before CG	Since CG
Strongly Disagree	Before CG	Since CG
Name(s)		
Comments		

THERE ARE PEOPLE I CAN REACH OUT TO AS NEEDS ARISE.

Strongly Agree	Before CG	Since CG
Agree	Before CG	Since CG
Disagree	Before CG	Since CG
Strongly Disagree	Before CG	Since CG
Name(s)		
Comments		

As you considered the four key elements of an effective SSN (companionship, confidant(s), intimacy, and conflict resolution), what came to mind? Does one person fill all four? Or are there several people, each meeting different needs? Which of these needs are currently being met? Which aren't?

HOW MANY IS ENOUGH?

The number of people and levels of closeness desired in your SSN depends on you. One person may be content with a few close friends, another wants hundreds of acquaintances. The number of people you need might change drastically because of caregiving. For the next exercise determine what groups of people are in your SSN, and whether it seems you have enough, too many, or not enough people in your SSN. Let's look at little closer.

EXERCISE: The Size of Your SSN

What Groups of People are in Your SSN?

Family
Friends
Neighbors
Coworkers

Members of your church
School acquaintances
Volunteer organization
Other

EXERCISE: The Right Number of People in Your SSN

I HAVE ENOUGH PEOPLE IN MY SSN.

Strongly Agree	Before CG	Since CG
Agree	Before CG	Since CG
Disagree	Before CG	Since CG
Strongly Disagree	Before CG	Since CG
Name(s)		
Comments		

I HAVE TOO MANY PEOPLE IN MY SSN.

Strongly Agree	Before CG	Since CG
Agree	Before CG	Since CG
Disagree	Before CG	Since CG
Strongly Disagree	Before CG	Since CG
Name(s)		
Comments		

I DON'T HAVE ENOUGH PEOPLE IN MY SSN TO GET ALL THE HELP I NEED.

Strongly Agree	Before CG	Since CG
Agree	Before CG	Since CG
Disagree	Before CG	Since CG
Strongly Disagree	Before CG	Since CG
Name(s)		
Comments		

Whether your SSN has only a few people or hundreds, it's important in the midst of caregiving that your SSN meets your needs for support. The questionnaire in the next section will help you clarify your feelings and assess your level of satisfaction with your SSN.

Gwen: Before my sister's multiple sclerosis, my life was filled with fun activities. Now, I'm too tired. I still get some invitations, but few offers of help. It feels like too many people, and not enough helpful people.

Mary: My husband and I have always been each other's best friends. We haven't wanted many people in our lives. Since his disabling car accident, we need more people. Is it fair to ask people for help when they weren't close friends before?

SATISFACTION WITH YOUR SSN

This section deals with your level of satisfaction with your SSN. Whether you have only a few people or hundreds, does your SSN meet your needs for support? There are 24 questions in the following exercise. Take your time, pondering over the questions, thinking about, appreciating, and recording the names of people who do fill these needs.

EXERCISE: Twenty-Four Questions to Rate Your Satisfaction with Your SSN

As you move through these questions, as certain people come to mind, write down their names.

I AM SATISFIED WITH THE WAY THAT OTHERS IN MY SSN DO THE FOLLOWING:

1. Encourage me to talk to about my fears and insecurities.

Strongly Agree	Before CG	Since CG
Agree	Before CG	Since CG
Disagree	Before CG	Since CG
Strongly Disagree	Before CG	Since CG
Name(s)		
Comments		

2. Give me information and guidance about caregiving.
    Strongly Agree   Before CG   Since CG
    Agree   Before CG   Since CG
    Disagree   Before CG   Since CG
    Strongly Disagree   Before CG   Since CG
    Name(s)
    Comments

3. Respect and honor all my decisions, even when I didn't accept their suggestions.
    Strongly Agree   Before CG   Since CG
    Agree   Before CG   Since CG
    Disagree   Before CG   Since CG
    Strongly Disagree   Before CG   Since CG
    Name(s)
    Comments

4. Offer to help me with tasks.
    Strongly Agree   Before CG   Since CG
    Agree   Before CG   Since CG
    Disagree   Before CG   Since CG
    Strongly Disagree   Before CG   Since CG
    Name(s)
    Comments

5. Assure me that I am accepted no matter what.
    Strongly Agree   Before CG   Since CG
    Agree   Before CG   Since CG
    Disagree   Before CG   Since CG
    Strongly Disagree   Before CG   Since CG
    Name(s)
    Comments

6. Truly listen to me.

Strongly Agree	Before CG	Since CG
Agree	Before CG	Since CG
Disagree	Before CG	Since CG
Strongly Disagree	Before CG	Since CG

Name(s)

Comments

7. Help me feel optimistic.

Strongly Agree	Before CG	Since CG
Agree	Before CG	Since CG
Disagree	Before CG	Since CG
Strongly Disagree	Before CG	Since CG

Name(s)

Comments

8. Help me get through today.

Strongly Agree	Before CG	Since CG
Agree	Before CG	Since CG
Disagree	Before CG	Since CG
Strongly Disagree	Before CG	Since CG

Name(s)

Comments

9. Give me information about how others have handled similar situations.

Strongly Agree	Before CG	Since CG
Agree	Before CG	Since CG
Disagree	Before CG	Since CG
Strongly Disagree	Before CG	Since CG

Name(s)

Comments

10. Provide the kind of support I need if I'm acting in self-defeating ways.

Strongly Agree	Before CG	Since CG
Agree	Before CG	Since CG
Disagree	Before CG	Since CG
Strongly Disagree	Before CG	Since CG

Name(s)

Comments

11. Offer to provide me with or guide me to financial assistance.

Strongly Agree	Before CG	Since CG
Agree	Before CG	Since CG
Disagree	Before CG	Since CG
Strongly Disagree	Before CG	Since CG

Name(s)

Comments

12. Take over some tasks for me.

Strongly Agree	Before CG	Since CG
Agree	Before CG	Since CG
Disagree	Before CG	Since CG
Strongly Disagree	Before CG	Since CG

Name(s)

Comments

13. Give me information about needed services.

Strongly Agree	Before CG	Since CG
Agree	Before CG	Since CG
Disagree	Before CG	Since CG
Strongly Disagree	Before CG	Since CG

Name(s)

Comments

14. Reassure me that it's normal to have the feelings I have about my situation.

Strongly Agree	Before CG	Since CG
Agree	Before CG	Since CG
Disagree	Before CG	Since CG
Strongly Disagree	Before CG	Since CG
Name(s)		
Comments		

15. Assure me that I belong and am cared about.

Strongly Agree	Before CG	Since CG
Agree	Before CG	Since CG
Disagree	Before CG	Since CG
Strongly Disagree	Before CG	Since CG
Name(s)		
Comments		

16. Assure me I'm respected, valued, and wanted no matter what.

Strongly Agree	Before CG	Since CG
Agree	Before CG	Since CG
Disagree	Before CG	Since CG
Strongly Disagree	Before CG	Since CG
Name(s)		
Comments		

17. Serve as models or examples for me to follow and look up to.

Strongly Agree	Before CG	Since CG
Agree	Before CG	Since CG
Disagree	Before CG	Since CG
Strongly Disagree	Before CG	Since CG
Name(s)		
Comments		

18. Remind me that I have a right to take time for myself and my interests.

Strongly Agree	Before CG	Since CG
Agree	Before CG	Since CG
Disagree	Before CG	Since CG
Strongly Disagree	Before CG	Since CG

Name(s)

Comments

19. Accept me with all my feelings (anger, sadness, despair, fear).

Strongly Agree	Before CG	Since CG
Agree	Before CG	Since CG
Disagree	Before CG	Since CG
Strongly Disagree	Before CG	Since CG

Name(s)

Comments

20. Help me set realistic goals.

Strongly Agree	Before CG	Since CG
Agree	Before CG	Since CG
Disagree	Before CG	Since CG
Strongly Disagree	Before CG	Since CG

Name(s)

Comments

21. Applaud my courage, commitment, and determination to care for my loved one.

Strongly Agree	Before CG	Since CG
Agree	Before CG	Since CG
Disagree	Before CG	Since CG
Strongly Disagree	Before CG	Since CG

Name(s)

Comments

22. Give me suggestions to cope with my situation.

Strongly Agree	Before CG	Since CG
Agree	Before CG	Since CG
Disagree	Before CG	Since CG
Strongly Disagree	Before CG	Since CG

Name(s)

Comments

23. Help me see positive things about my life no matter how bad things are going.

Strongly Agree	Before CG	Since CG
Agree	Before CG	Since CG
Disagree	Before CG	Since CG
Strongly Disagree	Before CG	Since CG

Name(s)

Comments

24. Remind me that I have a right to be happy.

Strongly Agree	Before CG	Since CG
Agree	Before CG	Since CG
Disagree	Before CG	Since CG
Strongly Disagree	Before CG	Since CG

Name(s)

Comments

As you were completing the questions, did other examples of "support" occur to you? Are you clearer about what support means to you, and ways that your SSN does and does not meet your needs? Journal about your thoughts and feelings, recording action steps you can take to increase the type of support you need.

CODE YOUR ANSWERS

Select colored pens and/or symbols and go back over the exercise, coding the ones that have some special significance to you. The following are a few examples. Create your own, and be sure to record your legend of the color coding you've selected, so you'll know at a glance what each color (or symbol) means to you (see figure 5).

Blue ● Positive feelings

Red ▲ Negative reaction

Yellow ■ Solutions that occurred
to me during exerise

FIGURE 5

EXERCISE: Overall Satisfaction with Your SSN

OVERALL HOW SATISFIED ARE YOU WITH YOUR SSN?

Very	Before CG	Since CG
Moderately	Before CG	Since CG
Not at all satisfied	Before CG	Since CG
Comments		

HOW MUCH CONTROL DO YOU FEEL YOU HAVE TO CHANGE YOUR SSN?

Very Much Control	Before CG	Since CG
Moderate Control	Before CG	Since CG
Little or no Control	Before CG	Since CG
Comments		

HOW MUCH OF A PROBLEM DO YOU CONSIDER A LACK OF SUPPORTIVE RELATIONSHIPS TO BE FOR YOU?

No problem	Before CG	Since CG
Moderate Problem	Before CG	Since CG
Little or No Control	Before CG	Since CG
Comments		

EXERCISE: Review and Color Code

- Review your answers in this chapter.
- Color code areas where you're not satisfied, by selecting two colored pens or pencils. Be sure to note what each color means alongside the exercise.
  - With one color, circle problems/issues that you KNOW HOW to resolve.
  - With another color, circle problems/issues that you AREN'T SURE HOW to resolve.
- Identify changes you'd like to make to enhance your SSN.
- Grab your notebook and write about insights you gained while doing the exercises in this chapter.
- Write down ideas you believe would help you get the support you need.
- Implement any change that will help you get the support you need.

People are more likely to continue helping when their kindnesses are acknowledged. Feel free to stop and call or write to someone and express your appreciation, or ask someone else to call or send thank you notes for you. As you continue through the following chapters, you'll keep discovering strategies for creating an effective/satisfying social support network.

CLOSING

In Chapter 3 you did exercises to become clearer about what "support" might mean to you, so you can strengthen the support within your Social Support Network. Let's move to the next chapter, where you'll create a Mind Map of your To-Do List, and methods for managing your To-Do List.

Conquering Your To-Do List

TRAMPLED BY YOUR TO-DO LIST?

I used to run our house like a charm and manage complex projects at work without skipping a beat. After months of caregiving, I'd become overwhelmed and clueless about how to stay on top of the increasing demands. You don't have to end up overwhelmed and at the wrong hospital, as I did.

This chapter will take you deeper into Mind Mapping, a creative method for managing your To-Do list, which you sampled in a previous chapter. Because To-Do Lists are forever changing, with new items appearing daily, I suggest you create a new one for this exercise. With Mind Mapping you'll find categories becoming apparent, with visual cues for knowing at a glance what needs to be done. Mind Mapping will help you move fluidly through the shifts and changes so common in a caregiver's schedule. You'll be ready when offers of help come, when plans change, or as volunteers come or go.

When I discovered Mind Mapping I was thrilled with the way that solutions flowed. I use Mind Mapping for note-taking and preparing everything from a simple trip to the store to managing complex projects. Once I got into the swing of using Mind Mapping, it saved me when caregiving demands were pouring in and schedules constantly changing. My Mind Maps became my "knowing at a glance," my way to keep track of the whats and whens and wheres of my life. The answers were right there, sketched out, when someone said, "What can I do to help?"

WHY MIND MAPPING?

Mind Mapping (MM) taps both the right and left sides of the brain, accessing *your* own creativity, and *your* solutions to *your* situation. Just as every personality is unique, no two caregivers have the same situation, resources, strengths, weaknesses, intentions, or needs, and

It took three hours to get him ready and bundled up for the cold. We inched our way through the snow to the medi-car, crept along the slippery roads, and finally arrived. At the WRONG hospital. I'd blown it, AGAIN! I was forgetting appointments, losing things, recording wrong information.

no two Mind Maps will look alike. As more information gets onto the map, the less you have to stress and fret, because it's all right there, mapped out by your hands and your mind; precisely yours.

Your Mind Map clearly shows where you need to strengthen your SSN and *how* to do so. Your Mind Map will help build one step upon the next. So let's begin.

EXERCISE: Mind Map Your To-Do List

- In the middle of a piece of paper write "TO-DO LIST." Then circle it.
- Draw spokes from the circle outward (see figure 6).
- At the end of each spoke write and circle whatever words or phrases come to mind on your To-Do List.
- When you associate a word with an already circled word, attach it with another spoke, write and circle the new word (see figure 6).

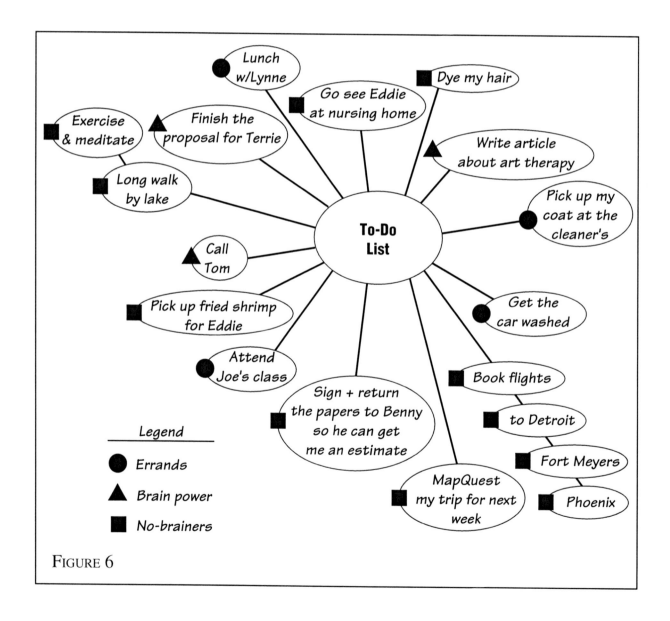

FIGURE 6

- Keep writing, pouring out whatever words come to you, attaching words you associate with words already written down.
- Create additional spokes if a word comes to mind that doesn't relate to one already on your Mind Map.
- Continue writing words until you feel finished, when you run out of words.

When creating your Mind Map, have fun. Don't worry. There's no wrong way, and Mind Maps are easily revised, rewritten, and adapted. It's from *your mind*. It's uniquely yours. Play around with Mind Mapping until it becomes comfortable and easy. You're sure to enjoy the creative solutions it reveals to you.

MEANINGFUL CATEGORIES

Study your Mind Map for categories. Look for new connections or associations between words. There are hundreds of different possible categories, unique to each caregiver's situation. You might have a different color or coding for each category, or for each family member.

Look at my sample Mind Maps (figures 4 and 6). Notice that *your* Mind Map differs from the samples. No two people will have the same Mind Map. Decide on categories that fit your situation, and what colors, symbols, or other coding will make items stand out for easy visibility. Use the sample Mind Maps to generate ideas, but when in doubt, honor *your* Mind Map, because it has *your solutions embedded within it.*

The following list shows a sample of categories borrowed from the Mind Maps of other caregivers.

- Daily chores
- Weekly chores
- As needed
- Things to do at home
- Things to do away
- I alone must do (such as getting my hair cut)
- Others could do (taking the patient to get his hair cut)
- Others could do, but I prefer to do myself
- I'm not capable of doing (such as lifting heavy stuff)
- I don't have the time to do
- I don't like to do
- Need to be done during regular work hours
- Appointments to be made
- Phone calls to be made

The Power of Color Coding

Once you've decided on categories, assign color (or symbol) coding so each category will stand out. Try this exercise to see how color coding works.

EXERCISE: The Power of Color Coding

- Wherever you are, look around your surroundings and notice everything that is red. Exclude everything else. Just seek out the color red.
- Next, look at everything that is blue, to the exclusion of everything else. As you can see, when your mind chooses just one color, that color comes to the fore, and everything else recedes.
- Select everything that is square or rectangular shaped, to the exclusion of everything else.
- Select everything that is round, to the exclusion of everything else.
- Select some categories, and assign colors or other coding for those categories on your Mind Map.

You can see from this simple exercise how coding, whether color or symbol, is a means by which your eye selects something appropriate to a given category, while excluding everything else. Each person in your house could have his or her own color. Things that must be done at home could have one shape, while errands that must be done away from home have another. As chores go on the list, and are assigned a category code, everyone will know at a glance who is responsible person for each chore, where it will be done, or whatever other information you've coded. Other categories might include appointments to be made, chores that need someone strong, a list for the visiting nurse, and so on.

Study your Mind Map, decide on categories, and assign codes to each category. Use colored pens, pencils, stickers, sticky notes, or whatever will help each category stand out from the others. At the bottom of your Mind Map put a little legend of the selected codes (see the legend on figure 6).

Where To Keep Your Mind Maps

The decision about where to keep your Mind Maps is also uniquely yours. Consider your daily life. Do you work outside the home and need to carry your Mind Maps with you? Are other family members or volunteers coming and going who'd benefit from having a copy of your To-Do List that is easy accessible? Would displaying the To-Do List on the wall or a bulletin board be best? Should it be near the door, near the phone, or near the office?

Consider some other caregivers' comments.

Kathy: My Mind Map is on a bulletin board in our office at home, near the phone, where I organize, schedule, and coordinate appointments—mine, my husband's, and those of volunteers.

Geri: Two big pieces of flip chart paper are pinned on the wall in the dining room. Everyone either passes through or hangs out in the dining room, and can see the Mind Map at a glance, what's on the schedule, what needs to be scheduled, or what still needs a volunteer.

Dottie: My Mind Maps are in an artist's sketch pad that I take with me wherever I go. I rewrite my Mind Maps every few weeks when they start to get messy. I carry the sketch pad with me, for easy access to current and old information.

Melanie: My original map is taped to the wall with hundreds of Post-its covering earlier completed items. I can look under the Post-it's to find things like previous doctor's appointments. I keep my Palm Pilot up-to-date with appointments, but my Mind Map has a fuller picture with key historical information.

Think about your situation and decide on the best place to keep your Mind Maps, putting them in a few different places until you find a place and a system that works best for you and your loved ones.

VISUAL CUES

Add visual cues so categories stand out when you scan your Mind Map. I had Post-its and colored labels, along with colored pens and pencils, for the notes on each Post-it. For example, a pink color Post-it meant that someone volunteered and it was confirmed. A yellow Post-it meant a volunteer was scheduled to help inside our home, and gave the name of the volunteer. A blue Post-it meant an appointment outside our home was scheduled, and showed the names of volunteers who would carry it out. Each Post-it meant a particular type of issue, with the names of the volunteers written on the Post-it.

With those cues you can see at a glance what's pending: chores that need to be done, appointments made or still open. Start playing around with ideas for color coding. Use colored pens and/or stickers, or create your own symbols.

Whether your coding involves stickers, other symbols, or a combination, the visual cues enhance everyone's ability to know what needs to be done, by whom, and when. Each coded chore that still needs a volunteer will stand out.

Here are some other caregivers' comments on visual cues.

Anna: I draw an image of a car for appointments away from the house, a house for tasks at home, a telephone receiver to represent calls to be made.

Lynne: I have some stickers with our names on them, so I could see if it was a task related directly to me, or one that was for another family member. With the sticker, each family member could scan the Mind Map for items with his or her name on it.

Suzanne: When a task was completed, I could reuse that spot by adding another Post-it. I didn't have to re-do my Mind Map as often that way. When something or someone was scheduled, including a volunteer, I'd also write it on the wall calendar next to the Mind Map.

Michele: I kept an errands list going all the time, so I could take it with me when I left the house, or could recite it if someone called and said they were coming over, and ask what they could bring. The worse things got, the more I needed to have a list handy, and be able to decipher it quickly.

Some people immediately embrace Mind Mapping. Others play with ideas about where to put Mind Maps, studying categories, deciding on colors, determining color or coding combinations, and choosing pictures and stickers. It's a powerful tool to ease the stress of trying to remember, juggle, or rearrange the endlessly changing tasks. The more comfortable and enjoyable the categories and cues become, the more control you have over your To-Do List.

UPDATING YOUR MIND MAP

Sharon: My Mind Maps are in a notebook I carry with me. I can see what I need to do and when. I can find dates or pertinent information from the past. At first I felt silly and somewhat resistant about Mind Mapping, until it shook loose some ideas. Now I love it.

Mary Beth: I keep my Mind Map on a bulletin board on the wall just inside my front door. When someone volunteers for an item, he or she signs their name to that item. I keep a current phone list pinned on the bulletin board and a calendar as well, for quick reference of scheduled appointments and phone numbers. Now communication glitches are rare.

John: Last week a friend noticed the phone list next to my Mind Map had lots of corrections scratched all over it. She left a note that she'd made a copy, and would edit and update it. The Mind Map alerts others about pressing needs.

Dorothy: I make my Mind Maps real big, on flip chart paper, so I can add names and phone numbers and dates to the items. I know who is doing what and when, and the contact information is all right there if I need to make a change or refer back. I also used Post-its for things that aren't confirmed, adding the contact information when I know for sure. When I'm not home others can see what's in the works and handle changes.

Ricki: I'm artistic and love creating Mind Maps. It's a meditative process for me. Ideas emerge as I doodle on my MM. Afterward I feel harmony between my internal and external worlds, calmer about decisions now, as happens when I meditate.

Find patterns, designs, or whatever coding works best for you, and as you continue to use that coding, reading your Mind Map will become quicker and easier.

SOME BURDENS WEIGH HEAVILY ON YOU

After I had that dream about being crushed by my burdens, I recognized that some burdens weighed heavier on me than others did. Some chores only take a minute, but are exhausting, like dealing with certain difficult people. Things I like to do are less of a chore than things I don't like doing.

As you personally think of stress as having a weight in pounds, give each demand, each unresolved problem, each unexpressed or unprocessed emotional pain an assigned weight in pounds. Then imagine each time you shift something, get some help, or give yourself back a few minutes to breathe, take a nap, talk to a friend, or have a good cry as an opportunity to lighten the load.

Try this exercise and see if it helps you put the items on your To-Do List into perspective.

EXERCISE: The Weight of Your Burdens

- Go through your To-Do List and code each item as heavy, medium, or light.
- Journal about whatever insights or feelings come from this exercise.
- Review the weights you assigned.
- Give priority to shifting items that weigh the heaviest on you.

By shifting heavier things, you can begin to feel some relief. Some things are heavy emotionally, other items might be easy to do but much more time consuming. What might lighten the load for you?

CLOSING

In this chapter we covered your To-Do List, and how to manage it. In the next chapter you'll identify gifts or skills of each person in your Social Support Network, so you can link the right persons with specific chores.

Nuggets of Gold in Your SSN

Love has a chance to flower in a shared life. Giving love is a fulfillment in itself.
—From the daily meditation book
One Day at A Time

FINDING THE HELP YOU NEED

In prior exercises you made Mind Maps of the various groups and people in your life. The exercises in this chapter will help you dig deeper to find people with the right skills, including those who've offered to help and those you've helped in the past. You'll begin by securing the vital role of "confidant." Then, analyze the gifts and resources of individuals within your SSN, linking people with tasks.

My world has always been filled with people like me, who enjoy caring for others. Yet, even when I was near self-destruction I found it difficult to ask others for help. A stream of people said, "Let me know if I can help." They meant it. If I'd asked, many would have stepped up to the plate. If only I'd had this book on caregiving, I'd have known how to reach out.

ARE YOUR SECRETS SAFE?

In preceding chapters you were introduced to the benefits of having at least one "confidant," someone you feel safe with whether you're feeling good or bad, happy or sad, with whom you don't fear judgment or a betrayal of confidences. The studies show that having at least one confidant far outweighs network size and frequency of contacts in importance for a sound SSN. Who comes to mind that you can safely share your inner-most feelings with? Do you currently have one or more confidants?

Deann and Lynne are my closest girlfriends, primary confidants known and trusted for many years. We listen, never give unsolicited advice, and never criticize. By being heard, we are empowered, and we feel safe enough to pour our hearts out to one another. Whether I'm happy, sad, bragging, complaining, whiney, confused, scared, laughing, or crying, their love for me endures. Without Deann and Lynne I wouldn't have survived caregiving. There were times when I felt as though I held them hostage as I chattered compulsively, trying to eject my pain.

Many caregivers have close confidants, special friends in place who journey with them through the harsh terrain of caregiving. Others were forced to find new confidants when former friends failed them. What if your best friend and confidant is now the patient? What agony. Losing your loved one, your confidant, when you desperately need to process the pain of his or her impending deterioration is an added stress.

Anne: My husband and I were best friends with three other couples for over four years. When my husband became ill, one of those friends criticized and gossiped about us, while the others stood by silently. I felt betrayed. It hurt to be losing my husband AND my best friends. I didn't want to burden my children, and my relatives were spread helplessly all over the U.S. With so much pent-up pain, when someone was kind enough to listen, I'd ramble compulsively.

FINDING A CONFIDANT

If your best friends and former confidants are unable to provide the support you need, start searching for replacements. Close and trusting friendships are developed slowly, often over a span of many years. But, the world is filled with people who are good listeners who will respect your privacy and keep your secrets. To find them, think about the traits of friends and confidants in the past that were important to you, and consider people in your current SSN who might fill that role. To ignite your creativity, grab your notebook, and create a Mind Map on "Confidants."

EXERCISE: Qualities of Past Confidants

- Create a Mind Map, placing the word "Confidants" in the center.
- Begin adding spokes and pouring out the words that come to mind related to the words "confidant" and "confidentiality."
- Keep adding words until the Mind Map feels complete.
- Who comes to mind when you think about confidants from the past?
- What qualities did past confidants possess that were/are important to you?

The following is a list that some caregivers might consider the ideal traits of a confidant. This list is by no means complete. Feel free to add other traits you consider important in your ideal confidant.

EXERCISE: Desired Traits of Confidants

As you consider potential confidants ask yourself the following questions:
- Will she or he keep your secrets?
- Does this person practice what she or he preaches?
- Is there congruency between words and behavior?
- Is this person reliable?
- Does she or he keep promises?
- Does she or he know and value you?
- Is this person comfortable with the expression of intense emotions?
- Will she or he be patient and kind when you're distraught?

- Is she or he a good listener?
- Will this person be available the days and times you'll need him or her?
- Other traits you need in a confidant?
- Do you sense you are being heard?
- Are the responses respectful?
- Do you feel valued?
- Do you feel understood?
- Have other qualities shown up on your Mind Map?

A GOOD LISTENER

Being a good listener is one aspect of being a good friend or confidant. Good listeners tend to provide unconditional acceptance. You'll feel heard, respected, and valued. Solutions surface, along with the power to set and reach goals.

The confidants of caregivers are not afraid of emotions; they are at ease with intense feelings. Releasing emotions freely, knowing you won't be judged, can be both comforting and very healing, while stuffing your feelings, or feeling like you can't safely share, will increase your stress and block solutions. Having completed the two exercises related to confidants, do you know at least one person you trust to be your confidant?

NEED MORE CONFIDANTS?

Do you need to add one or more confidants to your SSN? If so, compare your list of ideal traits to potential confidants. Talk with them. Do you believe you're being heard, respected, valued, empowered? If you're still not sure, test the confidant by sharing something of concern, something confidential that does not put you at great risk, and see if his or her response feels supportive, and conveys a sense of support, and you feel safe.

Some caregivers need more than one confidant, perhaps because of the intensity, enormity, or the delicate nature of some issues. Having two or three confidants allows you to vent your feelings without compromising the confidentiality of certain topics or dual relationships.

VENTING/CATHARSIS

During the time I was bedridden, I vented my feelings by writing and by sharing with my two best friends. Knowing that talking is healing for me, they listened. They didn't need to fix me, offer solutions, or criticize. They know and love me, and allow me to rant and rave. They know my venting for what it is, a release of pain.

John: My wife of 32 years has Alzheimer's. Each of her retreats into the unknown is another devastating blow. When I told my brother and sister-in-law, they snapped at me to "accept reality." I needed to blow off steam about losing my wife, AND after their reaction I also needed to unleash my frustration about such hurtful comments from people who didn't understand what it's like to watch your wife, your best friend and life partner, drifting in and out of reality, in and out of reach.

Jenna: In a gathering of our friends one night I blurted out my frustration about my husband's family, who wouldn't help but criticized and interfered a lot. One of the men in the group told my husband's sister what I'd said. I learned a great lesson from that. I had to be more selective. With trustworthy people, I could totally and safely release my heartache, instead of lashing out at someone innocent.

PROFESSIONALS AS CONFIDANTS

Professionals are bound by confidentiality. And many are trained to be good listeners. Sharon Mc-Carthy, the social worker from Hospice of the North Shore, was an excellent listener who never judged or criticized, never gave advice or interfered. Sharon's support was the most precious of many precious gifts I received from Hospice.

Individuals who answer hotlines at the National Family Caregivers Association, and other agencies, who are highly trained to provide services for specific illnesses, such cancer, diabetics, and Alzheimer's, are potential sources for venting. Facilitators or other members of caregiver's support groups often become confidants in a caregiver's circle of support.

Now that you've identified a confidant, or are well on your way to finding someone to fill that vital role, let's continue mining your SSN for other nuggets of gold.

FINDING TREASURES IN YOUR NETWORK

Get ready to Mind Map by having large sheets of paper (flip chart paper, for example), along with colored pens, pencils, stickers, or other methods of visual coding that you've found helpful as you've been practicing Mind Mapping in the previous chapters.

While you're creating this next Mind Map look for links between a task and a person in your SSN. Feel free to stop while you contact the person to request help.

I often doodle while Mind Mapping, sometimes lost in my thoughts. I discovered that doodling is like a combination of a mini meditation and art therapy, leaving me calmer and more insightful. As you continue Mind Mapping perhaps you'll discover what benefits await you. Play with formats, styles, and coding, making it uniquely yours. Now let's expand Mind Mapping, taking it to another level.

MIND MAP YOUR SSN

For this section on "Mind Mapping Your SSN," allow extra room around each person's name so you can add several spokes, listing pertinent information about each person. You can use the Mind Map of your SSN that you created in a previous chapter of categories and people, if it has enough space. If not, start a new Mind Map.

If you have many categories, with lots of people in each, record your Mind Map on something big, like flip chart paper, a roll of plain wrapping paper, or on a bulletin board where you can move pieces of paper around. You could create one Mind Map of all the categories and then create a separate Mind Map of each category. You decide what works best for you.

CATEGORIES OF PEOPLE IN YOUR SSN

So let's begin by creating a Mind Map of the categories of people in your SSN, including people from all areas of your life, and your loved one's life. You sampled this in Chapter 2. Here's my list of categories: friends, family, neighbors, coworkers, church, school, art community, colleagues in the field of addictions, women's organizations, support groups, volunteer organizations, community service organizations (see figure 7).

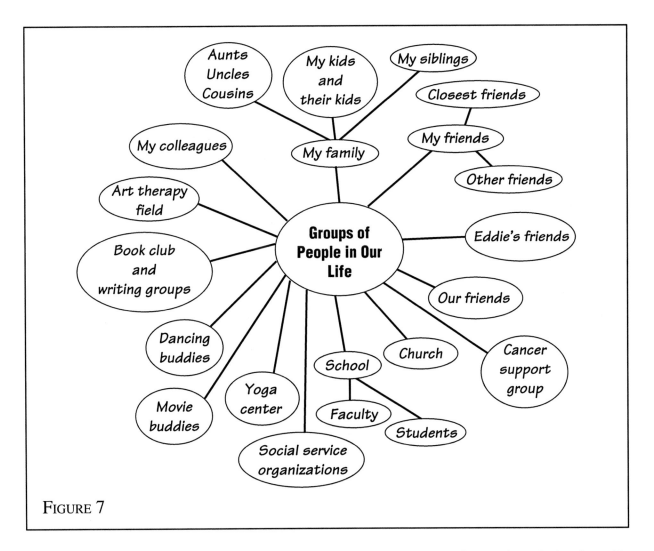

FIGURE 7

Because I have lots of people and lots of categories, I created a Mind Map of categories only (see figure 7). Then I created a separate Mind Map for each category where I have lots of people (see figure 8).

EXERCISE: Your SSN Categories and People

- List the groups/categories of people in your SSN.
- Then begin recording the names of people in each of those groups/ categories.
- Then, with spokes out from each name, list key skills, traits, talents, and qualities for each person (see figure 9).

SKILLS AND TALENTS IN YOUR SSN

What gifts, skills, and resources does each person possess? Would they agree with you about their talents? If not, what would each person say are their particular skills? One lady I know has a way of thanking, complimenting, and learning about others all in a few simple questions. She easily enlists the help of others with her warm and appreciative style. But, when I complimented her on being engaging, she looked stunned; she had apparently never considered herself "engaging."

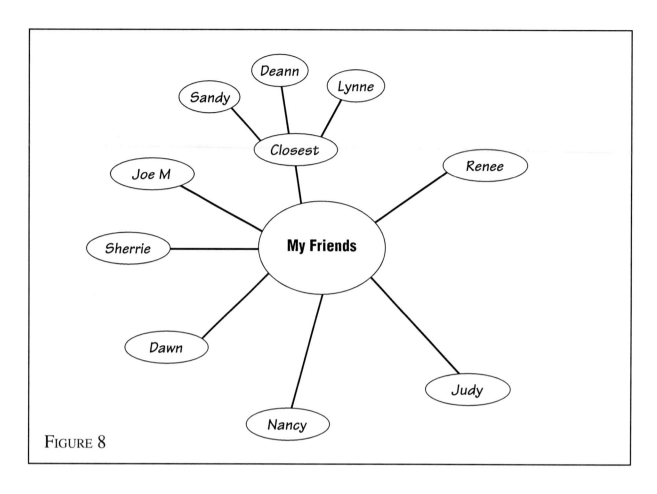

Figure 8

Many people are aware of their gifts, because others have complimented them. Just as many have been quietly going about life with a gift that others envy, yet they have taken it for granted or seem to be totally unaware of it. You probably have qualities like that as well. As you consider each person, what comes to mind, what talents do they have that you admire, appreciate, wish you had too? Let them know you appreciate their attributes, and if it's something they enjoy doing, they may be happy to help by applying their special skill to your caregiving.

EXERCISE: Unique Skills of Each Person

Identify key skills for each person in your SSN, including deficiencies that might affect their ability to be helpful, and continue asking yourself questions such as:

- What are his or her particular gifts, skills, talents?
- What is she or he good at, that you wish you could do too?
- What help has she or he offered?
- What skills does she or he possess that might be helpful?
- What drawbacks exist (e.g., unreliability, tendency to gossip, always late, too intrusive)?

Penny: I have a friend who offered to help. He's the sweetest guy, very well-meaning, but always late. He offered to drive my daughter to a doctor's appointment. He was 45 minutes late. The specialist, who was difficult to get an appointment with, was gone. It was a disaster. It took us six more

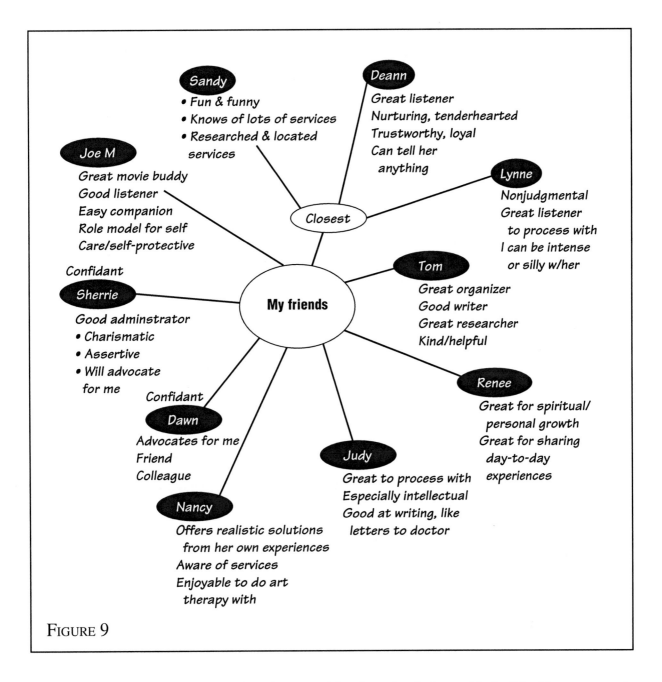

FIGURE 9

weeks to get an appointment. My daughter cried for days. I asked myself why I let him agree to do that, knowing he's always late.

He was gladly and graciously willing to help, and felt terrible about missing the appointment. He offered to set up my mailing list, made copies, and distributed them to everyone, so the people in the various areas of our lives could reach each other. Without a deadline he was fine. But, he was the wrong person when punctuality was important.

By recognizing her friend's skills as well as limitations, Penny was able to save a friendship and benefit from that friend's help. Think about the skills needed for a particular task. Some tasks require strength. Certain tasks require someone who is assertive or outgoing, or who has computer skills, or is well organized. Think about the talents of each person. Look for matches between your tasks on your To-Do List and their skills. Avoid linking tasks with people whose traits might cause unintentional negative consequences, such as someone frail being assigned a chore that requires physical strength.

People who are great organizers can take over coordination of larger chores, such as preparing phone trees and mailing lists, doing yard work, maintaining order, and researching doctor's bills and insurance claims. Assertive people can advocate for you and your loved one when you are distraught, especially when your caregiving involves difficult people and institutions.

Take out two of your Mind Maps, (1) Your To-Do List and (2) The people in your SSN. Study and compare to see who might fill a needed role. I was surprised to discover that I'd forgotten offers of help or hadn't considered particular skills of my friends until I began to study and compare my two Mind Maps.

When I think a person might be right for a task (they've offered, they have the skills, and are capable), I write the task next to the person's name. I call them, ask, and if they say "Yes" then I write their name on the To-Do List, along with needed information, such as their phone number, or an appointment time, etc.

EXERCISE: Linking Person with Task

- Select colors (and/or symbols) for coding.
- Record your legend for the coding.
- Write pertinent information on a Post-it, such as the person's name and phone number alongside the task they've agreed to help with.
- Some chores might have the names of several people who have the needed skills.
- If you're unsure of categories and/or coding consider the following categories and coding, if they seem to fit your situation.

Those who have offered help

Decide on a color or other coding to indicate people who've offered to help. Did they offer to help with particular tasks? Did they make a blanket offer such as, "Let me know if I can help? When asked to help (using their skills), they will likely say yes. If the task is not urgent, code it for easy access and contact that person later. If the load would be lightened for you by having this task assigned immediately (even if not urgent), feel free to stop this exercise and get the task shifted to someone who has offered to help, and who has the skills or resources to provide the help you need. Reach out and ask. That's the way to find out if their offer was sincere.

Those you can link with immediately

When an urgent item is a perfect match with someone in your SSN, stop and reach out, acknowledge their special gift, and request their help. You'll never know until you ask. If asking is difficult, choose a few people who are easiest for you to ask, then ask them to ask others for you. If the person with the needed skills says yes, code both Mind Maps (people and to-do) with the coding you've selected.

If additional information is needed from you in order to move forward with the task, make that a priority so you can get it off of you. For example, if Jim says yes, he will schedule Eddie's test at the hospital and find two volunteers to transport him, then get him all the pertinent information ASAP, such as the doctor's name, the doctor's order, the name of the test, the address of the hospital, phone number for scheduling, insurance information that's not on file at the hospital, etc., etc. By doing that right away it's another weight off you.

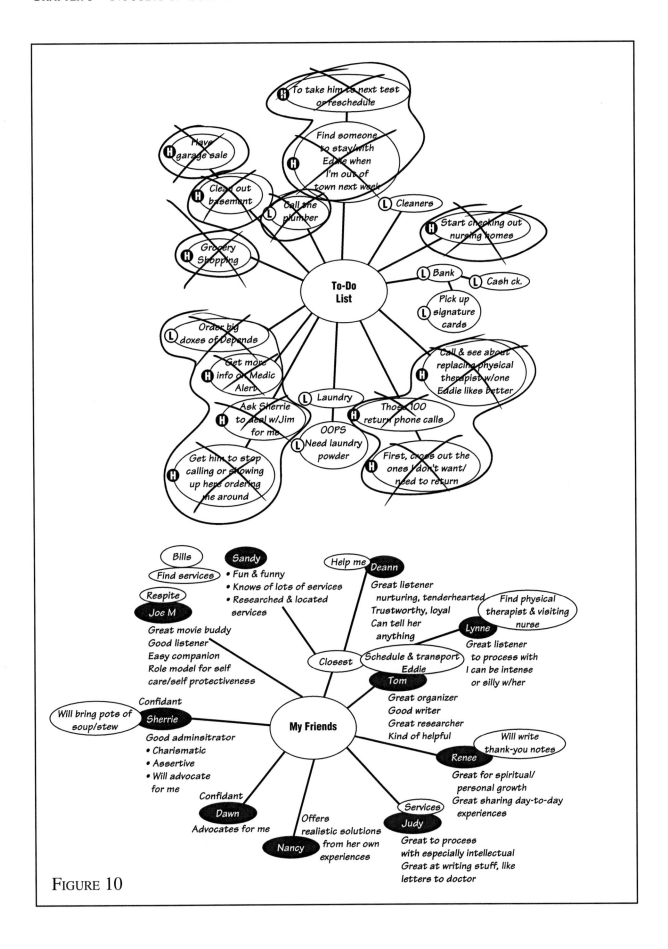

Figure 10

Each time something on the To-Do List is arranged, give a note to the person who has agreed to do thank you notes. Then, it's complete.

Those you can ask later

If the task isn't urgent, select a code and record the person's name next to the task, or write the task next to the person's name, so you can revisit it later, after the more urgent items are assigned.

Those who are harder to ask

Select a coding for those who are harder to ask. Sometimes you see a perfect match between a person's skills and a task on your To-Do List, but the person is difficult to deal with. Would it be better to have someone else request help from that difficult person on your behalf, or better to find a different person with the needed skill?

Those you don't want to ask

Select a coding for people you just don't want to ask. Maybe they'll help but would make your life more difficult. And it's perfectly okay not to want certain people in your personal affairs. Chapter 7 is dedicated to strategies for dealing with difficult people.

Tasks that aren't matched to people in your SSN

Do you have needs that don't match up with anyone in your SSN? Scan your SSN for someone to do the research and find the services you need. Someone who is good at talking with strangers. You give them the criteria for the service you need, and they can start making calls to find the service you need. You will be amazed at the services that are out there. In smaller communities, you'll be amazed at the creative solutions that emerge from sharing a need or requesting a particular service.

Too Many People in Your SSN?

Until my husband's illness, I loved that we had many friends and a lot of activities in our lives. After he got sick I started feeling overwhelmed by 20 to 30 messages on the answering machine every night, mostly friends and acquaintances calling for updates. I loved them all, but couldn't keep up with the calls. Finally our friends Sherrie and Jim set up a phone tree to reduce the calls I had to return, keeping everyone up-to-date for me.

EXERCISE: Too Many People?

Is there a person available in each group who you feel comfortable with, who could set up a phone tree and keep others posted for you, to reduce the number of calls?

EXERCISE: Not Enough People?

Do you need more people?

- What roles/needs are unmet by your current SSN?
- Who do you know who might know others to fill those roles?
- Who do you know who could make those calls and find some of the resources you need?

ELICITING HELP

There are millions of people in the world who chose helping professions because they truly enjoy caring for others. When people give of their talents and skills and their hearts, they feel good about themselves. Especially when the actions of the SSN are reciprocal, everyone can give and take as needed. With enough people, and enough resources, no one gets burned out. When people try to do things outside of their skills such as tasks they find difficult, they don't enjoy it as much, they feel stressed, and are less likely to keep helping.

Make delegating a priority. Shift something every day. Your survival depends on your ability to lighten your load. As more time becomes available, you create space in your day to rest and add back those people, places, and things that are medicine for your wounded psyche.

MINING YOUR SSN

For this exercise, consider shifting ongoing chores. Who in your SSN is willing, able, and reliable to take over some tasks entirely, so you can release all care, concern, or coordination of that task? In one case a neighbor took over a caregiver's car pooling duties for the mother of a child who was in a full-body cast after a car accident. The neighbor arranged to get the caregiver's kids to all their school and sporting events. The caregiver never had to worry about car pooling duties, until long after the medical crisis had passed.

The following exercise offers a few examples of items that volunteers took over for me and other caregivers. Add your own items to the suggested possibilities. Then, analyze your SSN for a good match.

EXERCISE: Scan Your SSN

Scan your list of names for people who do the following (if these would be helpful and lighten the load for you):

- Someone to extend thank yous—verbal or written.
  Search your SSN for someone to make calls or send thank you notes, so that everyone who helps is acknowledged and appreciated.
  One caregiver kept a folder where she placed notes about people who helped her. A friend sent thank you notes. The other volunteers felt appreciated and the caregiver stopped worrying about whether or not she'd remembered to say thank you.
- Someone to elicit help from others, if you're not good at asking.
  One caregiver found it impossible to ask for help except for a few close friends, who she feared she overburdened. One of those friends was good at asking for help and soon became the coordinator of volunteers. She continued in that role throughout the illness and beyond the death of the caregiver's husband. It's important that the coordinator of volunteers not take on other chores, because coordinating the actions and responsibilities of the volunteers is a complex and time consuming task.
- Someone to research social services locally to find out what's available, and what the criteria are for accessing the services.
  If someone else is going to do the research for you, give them the criteria. For example my friend Sandy, knowing that I needed a support group, with a sliding fee schedule, that it had to be at night, and I'd travel if necessary, found the perfect support group for me.
- Someone to take over some larger ongoing chores completely, such as the lawn, phone lists, shopping, laundry, car pooling, etc. etc.

When a volunteer takes over a chore in its entirety, the caregiver (or the coordinator of volunteers) doesn't have to reschedule the chore every time a change occurs. For example, a group of neighbors took on the task of maintaining the lawn. Several friends maintained phone trees for me. When a phone number changed, they corrected and distributed a new list to everyone, including me.

EXERCISE: Barriers to Matching and Shifting Chores

- Have you been able to match some people to some chores?
- What internal barriers have you encountered, such as difficulty in asking for help?
- What external barriers have you encountered, e.g., too few friends, limited social services in the area?

Keep a list of unmet needs with you all the time. When someone asks what you need, or how they might help, recite everything on your list. After I started sharing my dilemmas, frustrations, and unmet needs, I was amazed at how much help I found.

After analyzing your current SSN for skills and resources, were you able to shift items, secure help, and find additional needed resources? For the remaining items, take some time to journal about the remaining problems and potential solutions. Talk to others—family, friends, professional helpers—and keep searching for solutions to ease the load.

CLOSING

In this chapter you created Mind Maps of groups and people in your life, finding and linking the right person with the right tasks. Are you having trouble asking people for help, or in delegating? In the next chapter on Empowering the Caregiver, you'll find some helpful exercises to identify and interrupt limiting beliefs that might be barriers to getting the help you need.

Empowering the Caregiver

You Deserve Happiness?

As you read the caregiver's right in the sidebar, what is your reaction? Did your inner voice cry out, "YES, YES, YES!" Or perhaps instead, a weary, "Don't I wish!" Do you agree and wish the people around you did too? Are you plagued instead with feelings of powerlessness, unworthiness, hopelessness, depression, or despair? The beliefs that drive our lives are as unique as our personalities, with thousands, perhaps millions of unconscious beliefs influencing our decisions.

In this chapter we'll look at some common limiting beliefs such as feelings of powerlessness or unworthiness. Caregiving can wear you down, erode your self esteem, perpetuate feelings of futility, and prevent you from getting the help you need. The exercises in this chapter are designed to heighten awareness of your own internal barriers, and enhance motivation and personal power. There's also a section in this chapter on finding a counselor, with tips on preparing for and interviewing potential counselors.

Before and Since Caregiving

The words *patient, loving, fun, outgoing* once described me, but I'd become sad, depressed, angry, confused, and impatient as caregiving stretched me beyond my limits. Other caregivers also said they felt sad thinking about the life they lived before caregiving. Don't judge yourself harshly. Think of your negative emotions as signals alerting you about your stress level as caregiving snowballs, causing more stress, and more negative emotions. Being kind and compassionate toward yourself can snowball in your favor, because as you shift tasks and share emotional pain, depression and irritability will lift.

EXERCISE: Words That Describe You *Before* and *Since* Caregiving

For this exercise, go through the list of words and identify how these apply to you before and since the caregiving experience. Journal about issues and insights that emerge as you do this exercise. Use the following list of words to assess your feelings or perspective of yourself *Before* and *Since* caregiving, using this scale for rating yourself.

	Rarely	A Little	Moderately	A Lot	Extremely
	1	2	3	4	5
			BEFORE		SINCE

Interested

Distressed

Excited

Upset

Strong

Scared

Hostile

Enthusiastic

Proud

Irritable

Alert

Ashamed

Inspired

Nervous

Determined

Attentive

Jittery

Active

Afraid

Unworthy

Powerless

Depressed

Shy

Friendly

Sad

Lonely

Confused

Insecure

Confident

EXERCISE: Sentence Completion—Reverse Negativity

Go back through the above list and check the NEGATIVE words that apply, and then do a sentence completion ten times to get insight into the possibilities for your life if you didn't feel that way. For example, if you feel unworthy, complete the following sentence ten times.

- If I didn't feel unworthy I'd . . .

Susan: The first few sentences of this exercise didn't bring any surprises, but as I kept writing, each new sentence began to bring me new and vital information about the deep feelings of futility I had about getting the help I needed.

Mona: I was berating myself for feeling angry, confused and depressed. When my sister said, "The reason no one helps you is because you're so angry all the time," I recalled my mother used to do the same thing to me, so I tried harder to control my anger. This exercise showed me that being stressed out and overburdened was the reason I was so angry, and helped me quit berating myself, and focus more on getting the help I needed.

Darlene: This exercise helped me get off my back. I stopped trying to ignore or suppress my feelings. When I got crabby, it reminded me that I needed a time out. The caregiving experience, dreadful as it was, made me stronger. The lessons learned enhanced my entire life.

ASKING FOR HELP

Do you have trouble asking for help? Is it easier for you to give than receive help from others? The following exercises are intended to help you identify internal barriers to getting the support you need.

EXERCISE: Asking for Help

Answer these questions on a scale of 1 to 4, 4 being the most severe. If the rating would be different prior to the caregiving situation indicate that as well. Take out your notebook, and journal about your responses to these questions. Give examples.

1	2	3	4
Rarely	Somewhat	A Problem	Serious Problem

- Are you plagued with insecurities about asking for help?

    Before   Since

- Do you believe you're entitled to caregiver's rights?

    Before   Since

- Do you treat others with more respect than you treat yourself?

    Before   Since

- Do you treat others with more fairness than you treat yourself?

    Before   Since

- Do you believe that others have a right to a life of their own, but not you?

    Before   Since

- Do you believe it is better to take care of your own problems than to rely on others?

    Before   Since

- Does accepting help from other people make you feel like you owe them?

    Before   Since

- Do you believe that you shouldn't offer help unless the other person asks for it first?

    Before   Since

- Does just talking things over with someone else make you feel better?

    Before   Since

- Do you believe that admitting hardships to others is a sign of weakness?

    Before   Since

- Do you believe that "opening up" allows others to take advantage of you?

    Before   Since

If your scores are 1's or 2's, proceed to Chapter 7.
If your scores are 3's or 4's, proceed through the exercises in the rest of this chapter.

Self Esteem

People with healthy self-esteem believe in themselves and feel worthy of the good things in life. If others try to exploit them, their self-protective defenses will automatically come to the fore. Some people have low levels of self-esteem, often the result of a harsh upbringing. Others have a reasonable level of self-esteem that eroded as caregiving demands escalated. These exercises are intended to help you assess your own self-esteem and to interrupt the negative impact of caregiving on your own self-esteem.

EXERCISE: Your Self-Esteem

As you answer each of these questions, consider whether the answer would have been different *before* versus *since* caregiving.

- On the whole, I am satisfied with myself.
- At times, I think I am no good at all.
- I believe that I have a number of good qualities.
- I am able to do things as well as most other people.
- I do not have much to be proud of.
- I feel useless at times.
- I feel that I am a person of worth, at least on an equal plane with others.
- I wish I could have more respect for myself.
- All in all, I am inclined to feel that I am a failure.
- I take a positive attitude toward life.

EXERCISE: As Others See You

Imagine that people who love and value you get together and review your journal entries from the previous exercise. Review each item and imagine how they would counter your judgments of yourself. For example, what gifts, qualities, and skills do they see in you? They may have a long list of things they think you should be proud of, and things they appreciate about you.

For some people just recognizing negative self-talk can launch an effective campaign against it. Others may need to revisit events from an abusive childhood to get relief. Some need professional help, others do not. As you answered the questions, notice what you learned about yourself and what strategies might help you change negative beliefs.

I'd been raised to believe that my only worth was in serving others, a fairly common belief in women my age. I'd also become viciously independent, capable of solving my own problems and running my own life, thank you very much. Even as the caregiving demands were crushing me, asking for help was out of the question. I was on the verge of snapping. That limiting belief had to change, and pronto. So I created the exercises in this book and took myself through them.

Rita: When anyone else was in my house working, I had to work too. I couldn't rest, or sit still. I was becoming more exhausted and the demands were increasing. I had to grab a nap whenever I could. Scheduling anyone to come over felt more like work than like help. I was trapped. I needed help, but couldn't break through my need to entertain and/or work alongside anyone who was in my house.

In Maya's workshop someone suggested that I have a friend schedule the homemaker for times I'd be out running errands. Then the helpers could complete their tasks, and my home, my safe haven, would be mine when I returned. It was an immediate solution. Meanwhile I started looking at my need to entertain everyone.

BELIEFS RUN OUR LIVES!

Whether we are aware of them or not, our beliefs direct our lives, often subliminally creating havoc until we bring them into the light of day. As we become clearer about our negative, limiting, or conflicting beliefs, we can begin to change them. The less we are aware of our negative or limiting beliefs the more they run our lives, try as we might with brute force to change those beliefs. *I* believe that you deserve love, respect, and lots of support, but such affirmations are meaningless unless *you* believe them too.

I have a friend who says that if anyone else treated him as bad as he treats himself, he could kill the other guy and get off on self-defense. Me too. As my husband's illness progressed I gave up school, slowly abandoned all my goals, withdrew more from friends and social activities, and my usual healthy diet was abandoned in favor of fast food. Sleep-deprived and exhausted, I became steadily more irritable and impatient. But I had a belief that I should always be sweet, kind, and patient. I judged myself harshly at first. Slowly I got angry at demanding people, but it took much longer for me to see how badly I was treating myself by putting up with unreasonable people.

The following are some sentence completions that helped me recognize my limiting beliefs and become more compassionate with myself.

EXERCISE: Sentence Completions—If I Valued Myself

Complete the following sentence ten times, spilling out whatever comes to mind. If at the end of the ten sentences, more insights are still coming up, keep writing until you feel finished (see figure 11). Sometimes great insights come just as you think you're running out of things to say.

If I loved and valued myself more I'd . . .

After the ten sentences, if something negative came up, then also do the following sentence completions by taking the negative insight and completing the following sentence over and over. For example: If I was doing the sentence completion *If I loved and valued myself . . .* , and I wrote *I'd stick up for myself more* (which is positive), but my mother would say I was selfish (which felt negative), then I would begin a second set of sentence completions about proceeding even in the face of resistance (internal or external).

---

1. If I loved and valued myself more I'd set limits with those difficult people

2. If I loved and valued myself more I'd shift more things, so I could get more rest

3. If I loved and valued myself more I'd finish this book and get it published

4. If I loved and valued myself more I'd meditate on God's love everyday, meditation is time with God that always makes me feel better

5. If I loved and valued myself more I'd begin and end each day with a gratitude list, because that also makes me feel much better

6. If I loved and valued myself more I'd study the Course in Miracles everyday

7. If I loved and valued myself more I'd spend time with the people who love and value me, and stay clear of those who are hurtful

8. If I loved and valued myself more I'd be able to rest while others are in the house helping out

9. If I loved and valued myself more I'd go to Sedona for a time out

10. If I loved and valued myself more I'd stop berating myself for not being able to do all this work by myself

11. If I loved and valued myself more I wouldn't care what others think, or how they judge a situation like mine, that they've never been in

12. If I loved and valued myself more I'd ask for and accept help

Figure 11

See the way one caregiver addressed this negative reaction:

- *If my mother criticized me for sticking up for myself then we'd get into an argument.*
- *If I stick to my guns she'll realize that I won't let her exploit me anymore.*
- *If I don't let her exploit me anymore, I'll feel better about myself.*
- *If I feel better about myself and stick up for myself, then I'll have more time for myself.*
- *If I have more time for myself I'll be less exhausted.*

I realized as I did this exercise that some people in my life have taken advantage of me for a long time. To change that I'll have to endure some stressful interactions, but eventually if I don't back down, they'll back off, and my life will be better.

HONORING MY RIGHTS

EXERCISE: If I Believe I'm Deserving

Go back to each caregiver's right, which can be found in the exercise on page 8 in chapter 2. For each of the caregiver's rights that you have difficulty honoring, do a sentence completion ten times for each of these three items.

- If I honored that right . . .
- If I enforced that right . . .
- If I told others that I object when they don't honor that right . . .

Keep doing the sentence completions to see the payoffs you can expect from honoring all the caregiver's rights, and doing positive things for yourself.

When you're reviewing the caregiver's rights and identify a negative or limiting belief, such as:

- I'm too scared to stand up for myself.
- I feel too powerless to get anyone to listen to me.
- I don't feel worthy of asking for help.

Then proceed to the next exercise.

EXERCISE: Sentence Completions on Limiting Beliefs

Do ten sentence completions for each of the three limiting beliefs by pretending what it would be like if you didn't feel that way.

If I Didn't Feel . . .

- If I didn't feel scared I'd . . .
- If I didn't feel powerless I'd . . .
- If I didn't feel unworthy I'd . . .

1. If I didn't feel scared I'd stand up to hurtful people

2. If I didn't feel scared I'd be able to move forward with my goals without so much second-guessing and fretting

3. If I didn't feel scared I'd be happier

4. If I didn't feel scared I'd be healthier

5. If I didn't feel scared I'd be more trusting of God, and the unfolding of this situation

6. If I didn't feel scared I wouldn't react with so much anger

7. If I didn't feel scared I wouldn't be so controlling

8. If I didn't feel scared I'd live a day at a time and stop worrying about tomorrow, which I have no control over

9. If I didn't feel scared I'd believe in myself, and my ability to deal with whatever comes

10. If I didn't feel scared I'd look at how resourceful I am and at all the difficult situations I've dealt with and learned from

Note: As I continued finishing sentences it became clearer to me that most of my fears are unfounded, that I have proof from past experiences that God loves me, that I can deal with whatever life throws my way, and that I have become stronger and more resourceful as a result of difficult times.

FIGURE 12

Before my husband's illness I had a full time job that I loved, and I was working on my master's degree. I had friends, family, hobbies, and various fun and social activities that I enjoyed, including several groups with common interests—the arts, theater, book clubs, dancing, and personal growth workshops. My life was full, rich, and enjoyable. Sometimes things got a little hectic, but all in all I loved my life. I went from lively, fun, funny, and personable to exhausted, depressed, bitter, resentful, and withdrawn. After my husband died, I longed to regain my health and get back to my old life before his illness. That's what I was striving for and eventually reached.

IF ONLY I DIDN'T FEEL POWERLESS/UNWORTHY

In my exhaustion, I felt powerless. Berating myself for being bitter, I felt unworthy and undeserving of happiness. If you struggle with feelings of powerlessness or unworthiness, continue with this exercise to see how life might be if you weren't held back by these beliefs.

EXERCISE: Sentence Completion—If I Felt Empowered/Loved/Worthy

Do ten sentence completions for the following sentences.

If I felt empowered I'd . . .

If I loved myself I'd . . .

If I felt worthy and deserving I'd . . .

DO YOU HELP OTHERS AT YOUR OWN EXPENSE?

Born tenderhearted, I was a caregiver long before my husband's illness. In kindergarten when another child fell, or got hurt or yelled at, I cried and soothed them. Raised to put others first, I was masterful at denying my own needs, easily lost in caring for others. Occasionally I rebelled or resented, stomping my emotional feet and demanding, "What about me?" Then, ashamed for being so demanding, I'd settle back into mothering the world. Through my husband's illness I could see how putting others first was hurting me. But, even with a concentrated effort I couldn't control my compulsive need to care for others, even at the expense of my own health and well-being.

To survive as a child I had to put my family first. I noticed other people's needs and automatically filled those needs without regard for myself. One day deep into my caregiving experience I was carrying two big boxes of personal things, when I noticed a lady scurrying toward the elevator too. When the elevator door opened, instead of getting in, I balanced on one foot, using my other foot to prop open the door for her. She shoved past me, knocking my boxes to the floor, my stuff spilling all over, some inside, some outside the elevator. She pressed the button, and off she went with half my stuff. Stunned for a split second, then I laughed at what a great role model she was for self care. Painful as it was, those lessons helped me see that my automatic habit of putting others first had to stop.

Out of my frustration and soul-searching I created the following exercise, which helped me gain insight into the underlying causes of my compulsive need to put others first. The exercise helped me and other caregivers to slowly and methodically convert those harmful patterns into self-love and self-protectiveness.

EXERCISE: "Others First" versus "Me First"

DAY ONE

- All day today, look around for people in need—a mom struggling with a baby and groceries, someone looking for a seat on the bus. Hold every door, offer directions, help with equipment, carry packages, give money to the homeless, give your time, service, or advice.
- Take each problem you see and make it your own. Fill every need you see to the extent possible.
- Journal about "having" to help others, what you saw, what you did, how you felt, what positive and negative experiences you had as a result of the exercise.
  - ◊ Journal about any needs you just couldn't bring yourself to fill.
  - ◊ Journal about needs you debated with yourself about. For example, when one part of you wanted to fill the need, while another part didn't.
- After you've finished journaling, process this exercise with a counselor or other caregivers.

DAY TWO

- Continue to scout for needs.
- But, DON'T FILL ANY NEEDS today.
- Journal about your feelings and reactions to your experiences throughout the day.
  - ◊ How you felt.
  - ◊ Which things you wanted to do.
  - ◊ Which ones you didn't.
  - ◊ Journal about your internal dialogue, inner debates about the situations you saw, and your assignment for today.

For twenty days alternate between filling every need on one day, and not filling any needs the next day. Each day journal and/or process with someone else your feelings, reactions, experiences, insights, and internal dialogue.

NEXT PHASE

After twenty days, add a third day.

- DAY ONE—continue to search for and FILL EVERY NEED YOU SEE.
- DAY TWO—continue to search for needs, but REFUSE EVERY NEED YOU SEE.
- DAY THREE—THE CHOICE IS YOURS. Follow your feelings.
  - ◊ You can scout for needs or not scout for needs.
  - ◊ When you see a need you can fill it or not fill it.

Notice what happens. Journal and/or process your experiences with other caregivers or a counselor.

- What needs did you notice and feel compelled to fill?
- Which needs did you notice but not feel compelled to fill?
- Journal about your feelings, insights, and reactions to the experiences.
- Are you noticing needs less?
- Are you feeling compelled to fill needs less?
- What kind of internal dialogue accompanies these experiences?
- Are you judging or criticizing yourself for not filling needs?

Keep doing this exercise, alternating the three days, until you start putting your needs first.

Peg: I realized that I felt guilty, with anticipation of punishment, if I saw a need and didn't fill it. As I resisted urges to help, I noticed myself helping only if I was asked. As the fear of punishment subsided, I was able to say "No." I was amazed at how much my life had been run by a compulsive need to rescue others. Today, thank God, I have a choice about whether or not to help others.

*Rhonda: As I got deeper into the exercise. I started getting angry at how much others took advantage of me. How could I feel OK about myself when I allowed others to exploit me? I continued with the exercise and I realized that **I WAS EXPLOITING ME, more than anyone else.** I started to set limits with others, began asking for help more, and started feeling better about myself.*

ARE YOU CONSIDERING THERAPY?

The guidance of a professional can help cut through issues with greater ease. If you're thinking about a counselor to help you through these tough times, be sure it's someone who understands caregiving. In the exercise earlier in this book you clarified what "support" would look like, sound like, and feel like for you. Use the insights from that exercise to recognize if a counselor's style fits the kind of support you need.
   Professional support can come in many forms. Here are a few examples.

- *Caregiver support groups* are wonderful because you'll get the benefits of a skilled facilitator, as well as the friendship and comfort of other caregivers.
- *Online support groups* are great for caregivers who are homebound and/or in rural areas.
- *Caregiver classes* led by professionals often focus on particular issues such as Alzheimer's, or diabetes, are often offered through colleges or hospitals, and provide knowledge, research, and strategies. The support in these classes may be secondary to presenting the materials, but can be a great means of finding and understanding the resources in your community.
- *One-to-one therapy* gives you an opportunity to get undivided attention, and to discuss issues that you aren't comfortable bringing up in a group or with non-professionals.

   To find a counselor who understands caregiving, prepare a few questions, and interview potential counselors on the phone. Tell them you're looking for a counselor who understands caregiving, and that you have a few questions. Their responses to your questions will reveal whether they truly understand caregiving, and whether they can meet your criteria for "support." Feel free to create your own set of questions, but here are some sample questions that a caregiver might use to interview a potential counselor.

- Do you currently work with, or have you worked with, other caregivers?
- My loved one's health crises might result in missed appointments. How flexible are you about missed appointments?
- In a crisis, would you do phone or e-mail sessions?
- My sister won't help, but interferes with the course of treatment for our father. What would you advise?

- I've always taken care of others; now I need help but am too passive to ask. What would you advise?
- I'm exhausted from the endless tasks, the crises, and sleep deprivation. What would you advise?

Are the counselor's responses respectful and sensitive to the realities of caregiving? Don't spend your time and money teaching someone, ostensibly a counselor, about caregiving, whose style is controlling, shaming, or blaming. If the phone interview reveals someone who is condescending, or in any other way makes you feel worse, simply move on to the next interview. Now, more than ever, you need to be treated with respect, kindness, compassion, and words of encouragement. Continue phone interviews until you find a counselor who understands the reality of caregiving.

An unenlightened counselor might see your reactions as character flaws, instead of caregiver's stress. A professional who understands the trauma of caregiving will be able to see the resourceful individual you are, and who you were before. A counselor with an understanding of caregiving will offer meaningful suggestions to help you reduce burdens and guide you back to your more resourceful pre-caregiving self.

If you already have a counselor you're fond of who doesn't understand caregiving, tell him or her about exercises or insights you've found beneficial. Your sharing may help your counselor to better understand caregiving, and help you implement effective strategies.

THE FUTURE YOU

We've all had hard times in our lives that ultimately transformed us, made a stronger somehow. In this exercise you'll get a glimpse of yourself with the strengths, insights, and personal power that awaits you as you rise above caregiving challenges.

EXERCISE: Difficulties That Made You Stronger

Take out your journal and write about past difficulties that made you stronger.

- List some times in the past that were difficult, but helped you become stronger and more resourceful.
- List strengths, skills, and/or knowledge you acquired from each of those tough times.
- Consider how some of those previously acquired resources are or could be helping you through this difficult time.

EXERCISE: Seeing Yourself in the Future

Imagine yourself at a party where you are the guest of honor, presented with an award for your selfless dedication to the care of your loved one. You're asked to share a few words. In your mind's eye see and hear yourself describing how much better your life is now that you've taken control of the situation, are self-caring and effectively managing the demands of caregiving.

See and hear yourself telling your friends the things you did to get out from under the lash of caregiving, what changes you've made, how you've taken charge of your life.

As you move through this exercise, journal and/or share your reactions with other caregivers or your counselor. In this exercise you'll be imagining yourself in the future. Visualize and hear yourself sharing how the new, evolved, and stronger you thinks, acts, and feels.

- Give examples of ways that the "new you" is more resourceful.
- Give examples of how the new you is more self-loving.
- Give examples of how the new you has greater personal power.
- Give examples of how you were transformed.
- Give examples of the challenges you faced that transformed you.
- Give examples of what you learned about yourself.
- Give examples of what you learned about self-care.
- Give examples of ways you are more self-protective.
- Give examples of how much more resourceful you are.
- Give examples of how much more self-loving you are as a result of caregiving.
- As the party ends, describe your life, including your ideal day, now that you've learned to balance self-care with caring for your loved one.

CLOSING

In this chapter you were given an opportunity to empower yourself by exploring and replacing limiting beliefs. In the next chapter we'll look at strategies for dealing with difficult people.

Dealing with Difficult People

WE'RE ALL HURTING!

As Marshall B. Rosenberg so beautifully points out in *Nonviolent Communication* we are all playing out our own unmet needs. Looking though a lens of compassion we can see another's emotional pain. Yes, even among those frustrating folks who stress us out. Their actions make sense when we look at the world through their eyes.

Caregivers tend to be compassionate and tolerant of others, sometimes at their own expense. It breaks my heart watching caregivers giving 180 percent, putting life, health, and resources at risk to care for the loved one, expected to do the impossible, and criticized for not managing the mess precisely as the accuser thinks it ought to be done.

I'm convinced that when caregivers set self-protective limits with those around them, everyone benefits. The caregiver's stress is reduced, the loved one's care isn't contaminated by undue stress, and the stressful behavior is interrupted. The focus of this chapter is to reduce the "stress-causing-mischief" of others, whether well-intended or not.

Tracy: I was taking care of my elderly grandmother. Two cousins called to ask for various keepsakes of grandma's, refused to help, but kept calling asking for more items for themselves and other family members. After filling 25 or more of their requests, one weary day I told them I didn't have time, but would add it to my to-do list. They called me selfish, and had other relatives and friends call too. Each time I gave them what they wanted, the next day the calls would start again, demanding yet another item, going from requests to unreasonable requests, to demands, to out-and-out harassment, getting others to call me too. No matter how many demands I met, they kept asking for more. Finally I said "No." No more calls. No more requests. If I were going to survive I had to put an end the madness. They couldn't comprehend the endless crises running my life, and didn't want to. Their want of some photograph or knickknack was all that mattered.

"Anything that anyone does is an attempt to fulfill unmet needs."
—*Marshall B. Rosenberg, PhD, Author of* Nonviolent Communication: A Language of Life

Victim Blame

Tracy graciously gave her relatives the item they requested. Then they stepped up the demands and kept asking for more, becoming more demanding and more abusive. Tracy's story is an example of victim blame.

Victim blame is when people use the victim's reactions, real or imagined, to justify their unkindness. For example is when a woman is raped, and someone asks what she was wearing. This is victim blame. When a man is mugged, and someone says he was flashing money around, that's victim blame. It's not okay to rape or steal, regardless of what the victim was doing or wearing. Tracy is a frantic, sleep-deprived caregiver. Calling her "selfish" when she can't meet the unreasonable demands of others is victim blame, and must be stopped.

The caregiver often gets blamed for not being able to do the impossible. Doing the work of ten people, then using that criticism to withhold help or compassion, clueless about the daily trauma and plight of the caregiver, these are all forms of victim blame.

Many caregivers are tenderhearted and giving. I suppose that's how they ended up being caregivers. Their affinity for peace and harmony extends to everyone, the deserving and the undeserving. In an attempt to be "nice" or "kind" or "fair," many strive to find fair ways to deal with unreasonable demands. If that's you, then for your safety, survival, and sanity put a stop to the additional burdens caused by difficult people.

You Deserve the Very Best

Putting yourself first can be difficult, yet it is necessary in order to deal self-protectively yet compassionately with those who increase your stress. The people in your life exist along a continuum, from angels to mischief makers, with most people somewhere in the middle. Many people will gladly alter their behavior to become more helpful and less stressful, if you make your objections and wishes known.

Sandy Saved the Day

One night at a gathering of our friends, I was ranting about people who were making my caregiving nightmare worse. My friend Sandy cut me off with an impatient quick fix. I blew my top and left in a huff.

Days later I was ashamed about the way I acted but still trapped in a storm of emotions. At the end of a horrendous day, one medical crisis after another, Eddie was crying in pain. In the midst of soothing him, the doorbell jolted me. There stood Sandy, reigniting my anger. She said, "Maya, I have something to say. Are you in a place where you can listen?" Through gritted teeth I said "Yes," while thinking, *And when you're done I'll give you a piece of my mind you'll never forget.*

Sandy said, "Maya, I love you very much. Your friendship is so important to me. I know what you're going through is horrible. I see you steadily crushed under the pressure. You've given up all your hopes, dreams, and goals, your time, your health, your money, putting up with impossible demands. I know all that, but I can't stand listening. Give me something to do! I'll do anything! But don't ask me to listen!" She barely took a breath and continued.

"Lynne and Deann are great listeners. I'm not." She started to say, "I love you, but . . ." I burst into tears, told her how sorry I was, how desperately I'd tried to find a support group. But all my phone calls, squeezed between a thousand other demands, had been unsuccessful. Calling from work was difficult, we were so busy. Calling from home was impossible, with Eddie's crises accelerating daily.

In the midst of my rantings, the phone rang. The voice coming through the answering machine demanding payment on a hospital bill. I starting ranting about all the mistakes on bills, and me with no time to verify which bills had been paid by the insurance, which hadn't, and what we owed. Sandy said, "I could sort through the bills, verify what's paid, what's not, and get all that straightened out for you. And, I'll find you a support group. Will you let me?"

She knew us. She knew our lives, our schedules, and our financial situation. Sandy took a box, the size of a television set, jammed full of doctor and hospital bills. She organized, verified, and condensed it down to a box the size of stationery. After that I could easily verify bills as they came in. She researched and found the perfect caregiver's support group for me at the Cancer Wellness Center in Northbrook, Illinois. With all the competing demands I don't how long it would've taken me to accomplish those two tasks.

Sandy loved me and gladly helped, but she couldn't listen to my heartache. Listening just wasn't her thing. We were bumping heads. Our previously enjoyable relationship had been knocked out of mode by the catastrophe of caregiving. Her courage in coming over and speaking her truth saved our friendship, and burdens were lifted. I stopped unloading my heartache on her. Yet, by helping she got a glimpse of the ugly reality of caregiving, how crises ruled the day.

Too Tenderhearted?

I'm very motherly and had formed relationships where I nurtured others. Under the lash of caregiving, with so little to give and already running on empty, I had to stop taking care of everyone. This was a huge challenge for me. When the crises hit, many of those individuals I'd always nurtured were happy to help. Others, deeply entrenched in our old way of relating, found it hard to shift. Some became downright resentful when I could no longer take care of them.

Are others accustomed to your nurturing? If so, as caregiving burdens increase, others may object to the loss of your attention, and may try harder to get your attention.

The Path to Self-Care

Sandy helped me see that both ends of my continuum needed work. On one end I let people take advantage, making excuses for their behavior. On the other end, when hurt and angry I could quickly judge others as intentionally hurtful, even those who are basically well meaning. Neither "milquetoast" nor "resentful" were attitudes that would enhance communication or bring the harmony I desired.

One person's voice can sound like a nightingale, another's like nails on a blackboard, depending upon your feelings and relationship with each. You may know precisely what irks you about one person, yet you may be baffled by your ugly feelings toward another. The following exercises are designed to raise awareness, offer strategies to help you deal with stressful people, and drain some of the tension out of relationships.

Put Yourself First

You are the most important person. That might be hard to hear if, like me, you were raised to believe that your only worth is in serving others. But the truth is that when we lovingly add self-care to the mix, everyone benefits. I lost friendships, and later realized I was lucky they were gone. Other friendships were gained in the process. You are the most important person here. Do you agree? Are you ready to enforce that?

EXERCISE: Who and What Stresses?

- Who Are Those Stressful Folks?
  List the names of everyone you find stressful. Don't judge yourself for your feelings. For now, just list the people.
- Levels of Stress
  Look at each person on your list, then rate the level of tension/stress you feel when interacting with each of these people, and if the level of tension was different before and since the caregiving experience, note that as well.

NAME   1- None or Mild   2 – Moderate Tension   3 – High Tension

Before and/ or Since

You've listed each person and rated the level of stress. Select a few people whose level of stress is "mild." Take one person at a time and apply all the remaining steps. This process enables you to learn more about each person individually and the impact of these approaches. As you proceed through the exercise, you'll gain more insight and confidence. Later you can start dealing with the more stressful folks when you've become comfortable with the techniques, when some of your stress has been reduced, and you're feeling stronger and more assertive.

What Stresses You

Take one person at a time. Write a person's name in your notebook, and what exactly she or he says and/or does that you find stressful. The more specific you are describing the behavior or words that stress you, the better it will be to bring about changes. Instead of saying that the sound of the person's voice stresses you, strive to be more specific such as:

- *Her words, such as "you know you shouldn't do . . . ," sound condescending; I feel like I'm being reprimanded.*
- *He acts like our friend while he wiggles information out of us and then gossips to our other friends.*
- *When I ask for help, she starts to criticize me.*
- *I asked him to help me move some furniture and he complained and criticized me the entire time.*
- *He judges without understanding our situation, and won't listen when I explain.*
- *Her meddling has to stop. She called the doctor, pressured him to order more tests. A Medicar showed up one day while I was at work and whisked him away without me knowing about it. He refused the test because I wasn't there to explain what they were doing or why. When I got out of my meeting at work I heard all the messages from the daytime caregiver, the hospital, and worst of all my husband, who was terrified and hysterical.*
- *Her brother tried to convince my wife not to have the surgery, insisting it would only prolong her suffering. We'd already discussed it, she knew the risks, but she wanted to live. I was grateful for every extra minute we'd have together, and resented her brother for trying to guilt her into not having the surgery. It wasn't his decision. It was ours.*

If the person uses specific words that set you off, write those in your notes.

WHAT YOU'D LIKE INSTEAD

EXERCISE: What You'd Like Instead

What would you like from this person instead of the behavior you noted in the preceding exercise? Be specific as you describe the behavior change you'd like.

For example:

I'd like her to use "I" statements and share her own experiences. If she hasn't had similar experiences I'd rather not hear her advice.

I want her to listen to why I handled something a particular way before giving advice. A lot of mistakes were made because I listened to people who didn't understand.

If he can't stop talking down to me, I'd rather he'd stay away.

THE BEST METHOD OF DELIVERY

Through my years of training in effective communication I came to believe that I should deliver information, especially unpleasant information, directly, openly, and honestly, taking full responsibility for my feelings and my part in the situation. I still believe all that to be true. But, I also discovered that in my weariness, I couldn't find the clarity or the assertiveness to apply the strategies I'd learned. I knew how to, even as I knew how to resolve doctor bills or find a support group, but I was too exhausted.

Instead of berating myself for not doing a given task perfectly, I realized that I had to shed stress ASAP, whether face to face, on the phone, in a note, letter, or e-mail, or through the use of advocates. Though hoping for compassion, and cooperation, I was grateful for every speck of the stress that was lifted, even if it meant the end of a relationship.

As you consider each person, select the method(s) to help reduce your stress in the easiest, kindest, and most compassionate way for both of you. At times I've used harsh words and a loud volume to get my point across, later feeling bad about the way I acted. The goal is to drain some of the frustration, so you can handle the issues in ways that don't leave you saddled with guilt and regrets. Select techniques that feel best for you, and best for the individual person. Begin by creating a wish list for your own life, then extending those well wishes to others.

EXERCISE: Select the Best Method

For each stressful person, consider each of the following methods of communication and select the one that would be the easiest and most comfortable for you.

- Face to face
- Phone
- Voice mail
- E-mail
- U.S. mail
- With an advocate/ally present
- A buffer, someone who carries the message for you

WISH THEM WELL

After you're clear about what behavior or words you want stopped, what you'd like instead, and your preferred method to address the issue, take a few minutes to garner well wishes for this person. These exercises are intended to reduce the negative feelings you have toward others, which in itself reduces some of your own stress.

I offer two ways to do this. You can use either, or a combination of these two, or other methods you've used in the past to put yourself in an empathic and resourceful place.

EXERCISE: Sentence Completions of Your Wishes

Allow your creative self free rein about your wishes for your health, wealth, career, friendships, your loved ones, or things you'd like to see, visit, do, or learn. If at the end of your ten sentences your creative self is still generating more wishes for your life, by all means, keep going until you feel ready to stop. Do ten sentence completions using the following (see figure 13):

I wish . . .

Jot down everything you wish you could have, be or do in your life right now. For example your wishes might be physical, mental, emotional, career, health related, financial, spiritual, such as more money, a bigger house, a better job, more closer friends, a degree, less anger, more love, time to exercise. Just spill out all your wishes for your self right now in your life.

EXERCISE: Extending *Your* Well Wishes to Others

After you've completed your wish list, think of the person you are having difficulties with. See him or her in your mind's eye, and imagine you are extending your wishes to him or her.

If necessary adapt the wish to be more suited to the individual. For example, let's say you know that she has lots of repairs that need to be done, but doesn't have the time or the money. Then, wish that she finds a way to make her home the most loving, comfortable, soothing, and safe haven it can be.

EXERCISE: Extend *Their* Wishes to Them

Next, as you see him or her in your mind's eye, think of what his or her wishes might be. Perhaps you know this person's hopes, dreams, or struggles. If they've had health problems, wish them the best of health. If you know that she has a dream of opening her own business, wish that person a life filled with the resources and support to start that business, and wish that her business is very successful.

Sentence Completions of Your Wishes

I wish I was healthier

I wish I had more energy

I wish I had more money to purchase the services to make my loved one more comfortable

I wish I'd invested more time and money into my goals

I wish I'd started investing much sooner

I wish my closest girlfriends lived in town so we could start a women's group

I wish I could spend a long weekend with my girlfriends

I wish I had more time to be with my grandchildren

I wish I could go to Sedona for a long weekend

I wish I had more time with all my friends and colleagues

I wish I had my book on caregiving already published

I wish my book on Women Empowering Women was published

I wish my Master's Degree was finished

I wish I'd participated in the Art Therapy Facilitators Training

I wish I was already moved in to my new home

Note: As I reviewed these I realized that some I can't do anything about, such as wishing I's started investing soon. When you come across items you can't change, cross them out, and revise them to be worded in the present. For example, "I will keep investing as I am now, plus I'll step up my activities around reaching financial goals."

I can turn wishes into goals, by adding action steps. And, I can prioritize them, deciding which to work on first. None are impossible or unreachable.

FIGURE 13

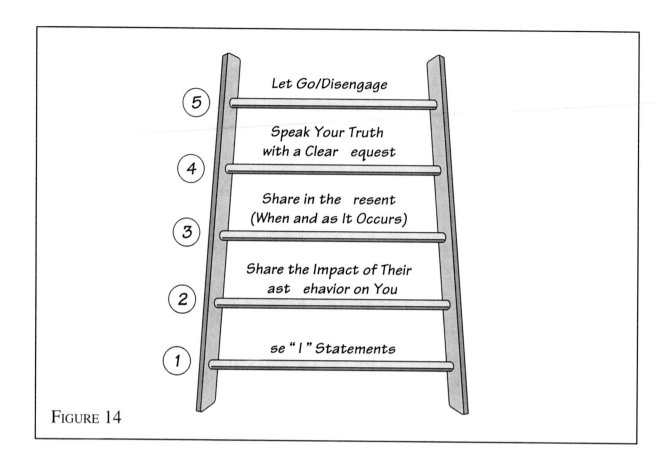

FIGURE 14

GOING UP THE ASSERTIVENESS LADDER

The idea for the "assertiveness ladder" comes from the manual on *Communicating Effectively with Health Care Professionals* (see figure 14).

The goal is to apply the right amount of assertiveness, at the right time, to confront the behavior or words that increase your stress level. Hopefully you'll be able to retain the person in a relationship that is devoid of stress. Mild confrontation will bring about the desired changes with some people. Others may require you to go several rungs up the ladder of contention and/or confrontation. And others might not be able to make the desired changes. When this happens, limiting your contact with those persons might be the only way to reduce your stress.

Rung One—Using "I" Statements

Using "I" statements, tell the person who causes you stress how you feel and what would be helpful, without talking about their behavior (see figure 14). Many people will be able to hear your needs, translate that into behaviors that would be helpful, and will gladly provide what you need. Don't be concerned or alarmed about people who can't easily shift their behavior. People who are not introspective may have little awareness about their own behavior, and therefore find it difficult to change. If using simple "I" statements about the behaviors doesn't result in changes, then go up the ladder and increase your assertiveness.

Rung Two—Sharing the Impact of Their Behavior on You

The model is simply sharing *"When people do . . . I feel . . . ."* This is still somewhat removed, but brings in examples of behaviors that have a stressful impact on you. For example, if a brother-in-law comes over to help, but while he's helping he complains about why your kids couldn't do it, or why you didn't fix it sooner, etc. etc. You can tell him that it's difficult for you to ask for help, and when others complain it feels like they don't really want to help, and you'd prefer they said no rather than resent you. Perhaps that will be enough said. If not, go up the ladder to the next level of assertiveness.

Rung Three—In the Now

Let others know on the spot your reaction to their words or behavior, including your feelings, wants, needs, and limitations. Behavior is the highest form of communication. True intimacy includes both individuals sharing how they want to be treated. The response you get shows you if they can and will be able to meet your needs.

Rung Four—Speak Your Truth

Do you know people who gossip about you, tell you what to do, pass judgment, criticize, blame, meddle? If so, tell them how you feel; be as specific and direct as possible. Ask the person to cease the behavior or the use of words you find hurtful and/or stressful.

If the offender's behavior or words persist then step up your self-protectiveness by pulling back from that person and/or finding ways to block the stressful behaviors that don't add to your stress. If you get their help and/or they stop the stressful behavior, that's great. If not, that's valuable feedback that they are unwilling or unable to cease the stressful behavior.

Ellen: My brother-in-law is a self-appointed big shot who flies into town and inserts himself into everything, giving outsiders the impression that he's in charge. He criticizes, bombards me with unsolicited advice, and tries to extract personal information from doctors, nurses, friends and family. And, of course, he won't lift a finger to help. I had to threaten the nursing home with a lawsuit if they gave him any more information.

Marilyn: My sister tells everyone that the problems wouldn't exist if I'd only listen to her. She twists every story into accolades of herself as the hero, and me as the demon. And, she hasn't even visited mom since the surgeries.

Rung Five—Let Go/Disengage

EXERCISE: Disengage from Hurtful People

After you've decided that you must disengage to protect yourself, apply any or all of the following techniques.

- As soon as you hear the voice of the hurtful person on the phone, say you're busy and hang up.
- Ask others to be a buffer between you and the hurtful person. Let someone else request their help and coordinate their efforts to help.
- Cut them off when they offer unsolicited advice.
- Don't engage in debates, just end the conversation.
- Start reading off your To-Do List and asking for his or her help.
- If you have caller ID don't answer the phone when the offensive person calls.
- Call when they aren't home and leave your To-Do List on their answering machine.
- If they persist in telling you what to do, interfering, judging, then you persist in reading them your To-Do List, until they realize that every time they attempt to intrude, you will request help.

Here are some other caregivers' stories.

Wanda: My sister said she'd help with mom if she didn't live out of town, but she promised that during the Thanksgiving holiday she'd sort and dispose of mom's old stuff. I believed her. She came to town, visited friends and other family. On her last day in town, one day before the movers were coming, she said she didn't have time, AND reprimanded me for letting it go for so long. That was the last straw.

I'd always included her in decisions about mother's care, because I believed it was the right thing to do. From that day on when my sister called, I'd recite the list of things she could do from out of town. I told her I wasn't interested in her criticism, or her opinions about Mom's care, until she did her part. Instead of helping, she started leaving messages at times when she knew I was out, asking for updates on our mom. As long as she didn't criticize or pressure me, I'd leave updates on her voice mail when I knew she wasn't home. We communicated through each other's voice mail. I would have liked getting some help from her, but the absence of criticism and pressure reduced my stress, so I considered it a success.

Penny: My husband was paralyzed in an accident. His sister made excuses why she couldn't help. She'd stop by, pick up tidbits of information to gossip about, and brag and complain to others about helping us. In reality she did nothing. I was running myself ragged to avoid putting him into a nursing home. When he asked his sister for some help, she said she was busy volunteering at a nonprofit organization. He'd always been there for his sister: often loaned her money, did minor repairs at her apartment, drove her places when her car wasn't working. It broke his heart that his sister had time for total strangers, but no time for him.

Caregivers share some hurtful comments, and possible responses.

- *I can't help you because I can't stand seeing him like that.*
  - If seeing the patient is too painful, there's plenty to do that doesn't include having to interact with the patient.
- *You'd get more help if you weren't so crabby.*
  - The caregiver is being blamed for having an emotional reaction to exhaustion. Do things that don't require interacting with the caregiver.
- *Why don't you make him go for those treatments? Or, stop her from having those treatments, it will just prolong her suffering.*
  - Most caregivers are compassionate people who want to help their loved one maintain dignity and quality of life by honoring their desires.
- *You don't know how hard it is being out of town. If I lived here, I'd help.*
  - Give them a list of things they can do from out of town and see if they come through.

CLOSING

In this chapter we covered techniques for dealing with difficult people. Whether well meaning or hurtfull, if their behavior is adding stress, they must be stopped. Put yourself first. Be kind to yourself, and use whatever approaches you find easiest to stop them.

Until We Meet Again

In order to get from what was to what will be, you have to go through what is.
—Cross stitch sampler on the wall of Maya's home

In the introduction of this book I shared my journey *into* the caregiving experience. The book is my journey and the journeys of other caregivers *moving through* the negative impact of caregiving.

I've formatted this book for easy access. The caregivers' stories are in italics, the exercises have a heading all in caps, and the non-exercise sections have regular headings that are bolded.

The caregivers who gave me feedback about the exercises shared their amazement that new things popped up each time they repeated the exercises. Like peeling back an onion, each time reveals another layer. You can trust that process like I hope you've come to trust your inner wisdom through this book. Each time you go through the exercises in this book, you'll gain the right insights for that moment in time.

My hopes are that as a result of this book you've created an effective and satisfying SSN. And that you have been able to resolve or are working on the aspects of your SSN that aren't satisfying. Some issues resolve quickly simply through awareness. Some deeper life-long issues take effort, but eventually progress is seen. Review the exercises and the answers in your notebook.

- In what areas are you still not satisfied?
- Has Mind Mapping become a comfortable useful problem solving tool?
- What else do you need?
- Are you shifting chores, finding the help you need?
- Do you have confidants to share your emotional pain with?
- Are there enough people?
- Are they the right people?
- Are there too many people?

- Are there enough goods and/or services in your SSN?
- Are you having trouble coordinating the offers of help?
- What else do you need in order to feel more satisfied with your SSN?
- What else needs to be done for your SSN to be more effective?
- Do you believe that you are entitled to all the caregiver's rights?
- Have you been able to deal with or rid yourself of troublesome people?

When I first began working as a counselor in 1976, I realized that when I work through an issue I automatically shared my own experience, strength, and hope with others. I discovered that I always learn from people I help. As you've probably noticed I repeated many times in this book that each caregiver and his or her situation is unique, and therefore the solutions much be individualized.

Twenty years or so ago I recognized the tremendous joy I experience by being a conduit for others' healing. My issue feels less painful when others are on a healing journey with me. While I'm in the thick of an issue (and I always am), I chatter about it endlessly, and I listen carefully to others' stories, fascinated by the similarities and differences, and the creative solutions. My sharing becomes richer as the body of knowledge, insights, and stories grows. My pain is eased as I share my process and hear the stories of others.

Somewhere along the way I also realized my spiritual mission and spiritual journey is to work through my issues and help others. After an issue is resolved it no longer sets off the pain, but when someone shares their heartache it fires off solutions, stories, and recollections of the wonderful people I met along the way because of that same issue.

Caregiving is a rough road, and yet it has its joys, its unique meaning. My hopes for you, the caregiver, the unsung hero are that:

- If you don't already know your spiritual path, it'll become clearer through this experience.
- The exercises carve a path for your burdens to slide out, and joy to seep in.
- By shifting chores you can create a space for the purpose and meaning in your life to manifest.
- By hearing my story and the stories of other caregivers you will feel less alone, more empowered.
- You'll know that somewhere out here in the world is someone who knows you are an unsung hero, deserving of all the best that life has to offer.
- You feel deserving of the same comfort and more that you give your loved one.
- You'll know that somewhere out here in the world someone knows how you make the world a better place.
- We extend love and compassion to ourselves and each other everyday.
- When you feel like you can't go on, you'll step around here and see yourself through my eyes, and see the wonders of who you are.

Wherever I go I meet people who are working on similar issues. Conversations and friendships form out of these encounters. I'm hoping that will also be true for you, and that each encounter will bring a story of hope, greater insight, new and better ways to lighten the load, making room for more joyful medicine for your psyche.

I'd love to hear your stories. Go to my website to learn more about me, and the schedule of my workshops. And when we are in the same place please come over and introduce yourself as a fellow caregiver. You are precious and important to me. During my caregiving I often felt desperately alone. Discovering I wasn't alone made it all so much more bearable. So when you introduce yourself to me, our world of caregivers broadens.

LET'S GET TOGETHER

I propose that at 6 am and 6 pm Central Standard Time every day, caregivers all over the world take a few seconds to imagine that we are plugged into a huge caregiver's pot of love. Imagine we're all holding hands, a blue/green stream of loving energy is flowing in and around all of us, as we're sharing and borrowing experience, strength, hope, and joy with each other, connected through this exercise to caregivers who need it at the moment, and for those few brief seconds we are connected together, millions of us caregivers all over the world.

- It is for you I wrote this book.
- It is my "never again."
- Never again for me.
- Never again for you.
- Never again for caregivers everywhere.

About the Author

Maya Hennessey has a powerful story to tell of obstacles overcome, and she tells it well. "My loving grandmother role-modeled the power of spirituality to overcome hard times. At age 13, when she died, I rushed to alcohol, juvenile delinquency, and abusive relationships. Catapulted into recovery in my twenties, I embraced a path of personal growth along with thousands of others, where I joyfully discovered my purpose—to help other women. Every woman I met brought insights that might otherwise have eluded me. Little by little the scars from my childhood were replaced with joy beyond my wildest dreams," she says.

Over a span of twenty-five years Maya went from volunteer to alcoholism counselor, to supervisor, program director, Executive Director of women's treatment programs, women's specialist in Illinois, and now a national consultant and trainer. Maya says, "Each of these experiences allowed me to cast a wider net and help more counselors and enhance treatment programs for addicted pregnant and parenting women and their children. When I visit treatment programs, listen to mom's stories, and hold their babies in my arms, my passion to help oppressed women is re-ignited, my mission makes sense."

"During my husband's illness I met other struggling helpers, and my passion broadened to include caregivers. I was fortunate to have the opportunity to participate in the National Family Caregivers Association (NFCA) on *Communicating Effectively with Health Care Professionals*, presenting the worshop to various groups of professional and family caregivers."

As the women's specialist at the Illinois Department of Alcoholism and Substance Abuse, Maya's passion to help women resulted in developing a statewide treatment system to empower addicted women. Illinois' women's substance abuse treatment system has been widely recognized as one of the most progressive in the nation. Her position included extensive public speaking, including testifying on public policy issues, crafting and influencing public policy issues related to substance abuse and women's issues. In 1990, in recognition of her influential role in the area of women's treatment issues, she received the prestigious Keith Keesey Award for leadership in Illinois.

Since 1976, she's been an addictions counselor, educator, consultant, and trainer and has served on the faculty and advisory boards of Governor's State University and Triton College. Maya served on state and municipal policy boards, including Chicago Mayor Richard M. Daley's Task Force on Women's Health. In 1998, First Lady Hillary Clinton and Maya met when Hillary came to Chicago to meet and personally praise the committee's work on behalf of women's health issues. In addition, Maya was featured in "Changing Lives," a segment of Bill Moyers' 1998 documentary series on substance abuse and addiction. In that series, Moyers highlighted Project SAFE, an award winning program that Maya managed, to help addicted families in the child welfare system rebuild their lives. In *The Counselor Magazine* in November 2004, Bill White, renowned researcher and author, named Maya among the women making a difference in the field of addictions.

Maya has been on CNN and PBS, and has represented Illinois in a meeting with Russian and Polish delegates to the U.S. Her participation included presenting information about empowering women substance abusers and their children, and coordinated the delegates visits to the treatment programs where families are being preserved or reunited because of the empowerment approaches of Illinois' women's treatment programs.

Maya's intellectual curiosity, commitment to personal growth, and passion for helping other helpers led her beyond the boundaries of traditional university education. As a certified Neuro-linguistic Programmer (NLP), Maya uses NLP to motivate people by identifying and changing limiting beliefs and patterns. She pursued training in group facilitation and leadership skills at Chicago's Oasis Center and has had additional training in lay ministry at Chicago's Swedish Covenant Hospital, where she served as an on-call chaplain for one year. Maya is currently completing her Master's degree at DePaul University.

Maya's commitment to speak out on behalf of caregivers embodies a charisma you'll see when you meet her. Maya's friends, colleagues, and participants in her workshops describe her as motherly, warm, delightful, and a dynamic public speaker, able to mix humor and humanity. In great demand as a presenter, trainer, and seminar leader, and a team member for training of trainers, Maya conducts workshops to such groups as the Illinois Alcohol and Other Drug Abuse Professional Certification Association, Inc., the Illinois Department of Children and Family Services, the National Association of Child Welfare Directors, Illinois Department of Corrections, Illinois Alcoholism and Drug Dependency Association, the National Substance Abuse Directors Association, and the Child Welfare League of America, just to name a few, and conferences all over the nation.

Maya plays a key role in educating medical and social service professionals about the links between substance abuse, child welfare, sexual assault, criminal justice, and domestic violence staff on breakthrough research on ways to identify, intervene, and refer addicted individuals to substance abuse treatment. Maya has had articles published on her work concerning women's issues.

Maya brings great energy and passion to her leadership role in the field of substance abuse, and the needs of caregivers. Maya's seminar's will be scheduled around the nation to such organizations such as Area Agencies on Aging, Hospice, Home Health Care Associations, and the National Family Caregivers Association to reach caregivers across the nation. Maya's website provides more information on her on-line classes and support groups, articles, books, tapes and seminars.

Before to her husband's illness, Maya says, "Life was pushing me toward the unmet needs of caregivers, in committee work on Grandparents Raising Grandchildren, and presentations on the topic of the elderly and substance abuse, and prescription drug abuse." The issues began to blend her expertise in chemical dependency and the issues of the elderly and caregivers.

Maya describes her grandchildren as, "The light of my life." She says, "Because my grandmother was a wonderful role model, delightful, tender, spiritual and compassionate, I share the joy of her love with my precious grandchildren."

WEBSITE/SEMINARS/BOOKS/CLASSES

My website www.mayahennessey.com is continually updated with my books, tapes, articles, seminars, classes, and training of trainers. My website has a link to reach me, and links to other websites of value and importance for caregivers.

My goal is to help caregivers organize their time, discover benefits in their services, find ways to improve their efficiency, uncover new forms of satisfaction, and exorcise the demons of time demands. I hope I've accomplished that through Maya's Model. I'd love to hear your stories, ideas, what works, what doesn't, and suggestions to make this book more user-friendly, easier to understand and apply.

Index

Resources

REFERENCES AND RECOMMENDED READING

Antonucci, Toni. (1985). Social support: Theoretical advances, recent findings and pressing issues. In I. Sarason and B. Sarason (Eds.), *Social Support: Theory, Research, and Applications*, pp. 21–37. Dordrecht, The Netherlands: Martinus Nijhoff.

Antonucci, Toni C., and Akiyama, H. (1987). An examination of sex differences in social support among older men and women. *Sex Roles* 17:737–749.

Antonucci, Toni, Fuhrer, R., and Jackson, J. (1990). Social support and reciprocity: A cross-ethnic and cross-national perspective. *Journal of Social and Personal Relationships* 7(4):519–530.

Antonucci, Toni, and House, J. S. (1983, April). Health and social support among the elderly. Paper presented at the annual meeting of the American Sociological Society, Detroit. MI.

Arling, Greg. (1976). The elderly widow and her family, neighbors and friends. *Journal of Marriage and the Family* 38:757–768.

Bloch, Annette, and Bloch, Richard. (1992). *Guide for Cancer Supporters*. Kansas City, Missouri: R.A.Bloch Cancer Foundation.

Brown, Stephen. D., Brady, Theresa, Lent, Robert W., Wolfert, Jenny, and Hall, Sheila. (1987). Perceived social support among college students: Three studies of the psychometric characteristics and counseling uses of the social support inventory. *Journal of Counseling Psychology* 34(3):337–354.

Burgio, M. R., and Tyranski, M. (1988, November). Comparing the social support systems and friendship expectancies of young adults and older adults. Paper presented at the annual meeting of the Gerontological Society, San Francisco, CA.

Cobb, J. (1976). Social support as a moderator of life stress. *Psychosomatic Medicine* 38:300–314.

Colvin, Jan, Chenoweth, Lillian, Bold, Mary, and Harding, Cheryl. (2004). Caregivers of older adults: Advantages/disadvantages of Internet based social support. *Family Relations* 53(1):49–58.

Conner, Karen A., Powers, Edward A., and Butena, Gordon. L. (1979). Social interaction and life satisfaction: An empirical assessment of late-life patterns. *Journal of Gerontology* 34:116–121.

Cutrona, Carolyn E. (1982). Transition to college: Loneliness and the process of social adjustment. In L. A. Peplau and D. Perlman (Eds.), *Loneliness: A Sourcebook of Current Theory, Research and Therapy*, pp. 291–309. New York: Wiley.

D'Attilio, John. P., Campbell, Brian, Lubold, Pierre, and Jacobson, Tania. (1992). Social support and suicide potential: Preliminary findings for adolescent populations. *Psychological Reports* 70(1):76–78.

Dean, Alfred, and Ensel, Walter M. (1982). Modelling social support, life events, competence and depression in the context of age and sex. *Journal of Community Psychology* 10:392–408.

Elliott, Timothy R., and Gramling, Sandy E. (1990). Personal assertiveness and effects of social support on college students. *Journal of Counseling Psychology* 37(4):427–436.

Felsten, Gary, and Wilcox, Kathy. (1992). Influences of stress and situation-specific mastery beliefs and satisfaction with social support on well-being and academic performance. *Psychological Reports* 70(1):291–304.

Fisher, J. D., DePaulo, B. M., and Nadler, A. (1981). Extending altruism beyond the altruistic act: The mixed effects of aid on the help recipient. In J. P. Rushton and R. M. Sorrentino (Eds.), *Altruism and Helping Behavior: Social, Personality and Developmental Perspectives*, pp. 367–422. Hillsdale, NJ: Erlbaum.

Fisher, J. D., Goff, B. A., Nadler, A., and Chinsky, J. M. (1988). Social psychological influences on help-seeking and support from peers. In B. H. Gottlieb (Ed.), *Marshalling Social Support: Formats, Processes, and Effects*, pp. 267–304. Newbury Park, CA: Sage.

Fletcher, Jerry L. (1993). *Patterns of High Performance: Discovering Ways People Work Best.* San Francisco. Berrett-Koehler Publishers, Inc.

Floyd, Maita. (1992). *Caretakers: The Forgotten People*. Phoenix, AZ: Eskualdun Publishers.

Garrity, T. F., and Ries, J. B. (1985). Health status as a mediating factor in the life change-academic performance relationship. *Journal of Human Stress* 118–124.

Garvy, Helen. (1995). *Coping with Illness*. Los Gatos, CA: Shire Press.

Gottlieb, Benjamin H. (1981). *Social Networks and Social Support*. Beverly Hills, CA: Sage.

Gottlieb, Benjamin H. (1983). *Social Support Strategies: Guidelines for Mental Health Practice*. Beverly Hills, CA: Sage.

Gottlieb, Benjamin H. (1985). Social networks and social support: An overview with research, practice, and policy implications. *Health Education Quarterly* 12:5–22.

Gottlieb, Benjamin H. (1987). Using social support to protect and promote health. *Journal of Primary Prevention* 8:49–70.

Haigler, David H., Mims, Kathryn B., and Nottingham, Jack A. (1998). *Caring for You, Caring for Me*. Athens, GA: Rosalyn Carter Institute.

Hirdes, John P., and Strain, Laurel A. (1995). The balance of exchange in instrumental support with network members outside the household. *Journal of Gerontology, Social Sciences* 50(3):S134–S142.

Hirsh, B. J. (1979). Psychological dimensions of social networks: A multimethod analysis. *American Journal of Community Psychology* 7(3):263–277.

Horne, Jo. (1991). *A Survival Guide for Family Caregivers*. Minneapolis, MN: CompCare Publishers.

Jackson, Billie. (1993). *The Caregiver's Roller Coaster*. Chicago: Loyola Press.

Jemmott, John B., and Magliore, Kim. (1988). Academic stress, social support and secretory immunglobulin A. *Journal of Personality and Social Psychology* 55:803–810.

Jones, W. H., Cavert, C. W., Snider, R. L., and Bruce, T. (1985). Relational stress: An analysis of situations and events associated with loneliness. In S. Duck and D. Perlman (Eds.), *Sage Series in Personal Relationships*, Vol. 1. London: Sage.

Kahn, R. L., and Antonucci, T. C. (1984). Social supports of the elderly: Family/friends/professionals. Final report to the National Institute on Aging. No. AG01632.

Kiecolt-Glaser, Janice K., Marucha, Phillip T., Atkinson, Cathie, and Glaser, Ronald. (2001). Hypnosis as a modulator of cellular immune dysregulation during acute stress. *Journal of Consulting & Clinical Psychology* 69(4):674–683.

Kiecolt-Glaser, Janice K., and Glaser, Ronald. (1999). Chronic stress and mortality among older adults. JAMA: *Journal of the American Medical Association* 282(23):2259.

Kiecolt-Glaser, Janice K., Marucha, Phillip T., Malarkey, William B., Mercado, Ana M., and Glaser, Ronald. (1995). Slowing of wound healing by psychological stress. *The Lancet* 346:1194.

Lakey, Brian, and Cassady, Patricia, B. (1990). Cognitive processes in perceived social support. *Journal of Personality and Social Psychology* 59:337–343.

Lapsley, Daniel K., Rice, Kenneth G., and Shadid, G. E. (1989). Psychological separation and adjustment to college. *Journal of Counseling Psychology* 36:286–294.

Lefcourt, H. M. (1985). Intimacy, social support and locus of control as moderators of stress. In I. Sarason and B. Sarason (Eds.), *Social Support: Theory, Research and Applications*, pp. 155–172. Dordecht, The Netherlands: Martimus Nijhoff.

Levy, L. H. (1979). Processes and activities in groups. In M. A. Lieberman, L. D. Borman, & Associates (Eds.), *Self-Help Groups for Coping with Stress*. San Francisco, CA: Jossey-Bass.

Lewin, Kurt. (1938). *The Conceptual Representation and Measurement of Psychological Forces*. Durham, NC: Duke University Press.

Lin, Nan, Ensel, Walter M., Simone, Ronald S., and Kuo, Wen. (1979). Social support, stressful life events and illness: A model and empirical test. *Journal of Health and Social Behavior* 20:108–119.

Mace, Nancy, and Rabins, Peter. (1981). *The 36-Hour Day*. New York: Warner Books.

Mallinkrodt, Brent. (1989). Social support and the effectiveness of group therapy. *Journal of Counseling Psychology* 36(2):170–175.

Morris, Laurel, and Montgomery, Bob. (1989). *Surviving: Coping with Life Crisis*. Tucson, AZ: Fisher Books.

National Family Caregivers Association/National Alliance for Caregiving. (2002). *Communicating Effectively with Health Care Professionals*. Kensington, MD: National Family Caregivers Association.

O'Connor, Deborah L. (2002). Toward empowerment: ReVisioning family support groups. *Social Work Groups* 25(4):20–37.

Okun, Morris A., Sandler, Irwin N., and Baumann, D. J. (1988). Buffer and booster effects as event-support transactions. *American Journal of Community Psychology* 16:435–449.

Pearlin, Leonard I. (1985). Life strains and psychological distress among adults. In A. Monat and R. S. Lazarus (Eds.), *Stress and Coping: An Anthology*, pp. 192–207. New York: Columbia University Press.

Peplau, Letitia Anne. (1985). Loneliness research: Basic concepts and findings. In I. Sarason and B. Sarason (Eds.), *Social Support: Theory, Research and Applications*, pp. 269–286. Dordrecht, The Netherlands: Martinus Nijhoff.

Portney, Dennis. (1996). *Overextended and Undernourished: A Self Care Guide for People in Helping Roles.* Minneapolis, MN: The Johnson Institute.

Richter, Stephanie S., Brown, Sandra A., and Mott, Mariam A. (1991). The impact of social support and self-esteem on adolescent substance abuse treatment outcome. *Journal of Substance Abuse* 3(4):371–385.

Robbins, Steven B., Herrick Stephen M., and Lese, Karen P. (1993). Interactions between goal instability and social support on college freshman adjustment. *Journal of Counseling and Development* 71:343–348.

Rooney, Brian. (1995). Evaluation of a theory-based intervention to satisfaction with social support. Doctoral dissertation, Loyola University, Chicago, Il. Available in *Dissertation Abstracts International* 56, no. 01B,0568.

Rosenberg, Marshall B. (2003). *Nonviolent Communication: A Language of Life.* Encinitas, CA: Puddle Dancer Press.

Sandler, Irwin, N., and Barrera, M. (1984). Assessing the effects of social support. *American Journal of Community Psychology* 12(1):37–52.

Sandler, Irwin N., and Lakey, B. (1982). Locus of control as a stress moderator: The role of control perceptions and social support. *American Journal of Community Psychology* 10:65–80.

Satir, Virginia. (1975). *Self Esteem.* Berkeley, CA: Celestial Arts.

Shaver, Phillip, and Burhmester, D. (1983). Loneliness sex-role orientation and group life: A social needs perspective. In P. B. Paulus (Ed.), *Basic Group Processes.* New York: Springer-Verlag.

Shaver, Phillip, Furman, Walter, and Burhmester, D. (1985). Transition to college: Network changes, social skills and loneliness. In S. Duck and D. Perlman (Eds.) *Understanding Personal Relationships: An Interdisciplinary Approach*, pp. 193–219. London: Sage.

Smith, Doug. (1994). *The Tao of Dying.* Stanton Park, Washington, DC: Caring Publications.

Smith, Manuel J. (1975). *When I Say No, I Feel Guilty.* New York: Bantam Books.

Stokes, Joseph, P. (1983). Predicting satisfaction with social support from social network structure. *American Journal of Community Psychology* 11(2):141–152.

Sykes, Israel J., and Eden, D. (1985). Transitional stress, social support, and psychological strain. *Journal of Occupational Behavior* 6(4):293–298.

Tennen, Howard, and Herzberger, Sharon. (1987). Depression, self-esteem, and the absence of self-protective attributional biases. *Journal of Personality and Social Psychology* 52(1):72–80.

Thoits, Peggy A. (1982). Life stress, social support and psychological vulnerability: Epidemiological considerations. *Journal of Community Psychology* 10:341–362.

Thoits, Peggy A. (1985). Social support and psychological well-being: Theoretical possibilities. In I. Sarason and B. Sarason (Eds.), *Social Support: Theory, Research and Applications*, pp. 51–72. Dordrecht, The Netherlands: Martinus Nijhoff.

Thoits, Peggy A. (1986). Social support as coping assistance. *Journal of Consulting and Clinical Psychology* 54:416–423.

Turner, R. Jay. (1981). Social support as a contingency in psychological well-being. *Journal of Health and Social Behavior* 22:357–367.

Vaus, Alan. (1988). *Social Support: Theory, Research and Intervention.* New York: Praeger.

Vaux, Alan, and Athanassopoulou, M. (1987). Social support appraisals and network resources. *American Journal of Community Psychology* 15:537–556.

Wandersman, Lois, Wandersman, Abraham, and Kahn, Stephen. (1980). Social support in the transition to parenthood. *Journal of Community Psychology* 8:332–342.

Weir, Renee M., and Okun, Morris A. (1989). Social support, positive college events, and college satisfaction: Evidence for boosting effects. *Journal of Applied Social Psychology* 19(9):758–771.

Winslow, B. W. (2003). Family caregiver's experiences with community services: a qualitative analysis. *Public Health Nursing* 20(5):341–348.

Wolgemuth, Elaine, and Betz, Nancy E. (1991). Gender as a moderator of the relationships of stress and social support to physical health in college students. *Journal of Counseling Psychology* 38(3):367–374.

Resource List

National Association of Area Agencies on Aging
1730 Rhode Island Ave., NW, Suite 1200
Washington, DC 20036
202-872-0888
202-872-0057
www.n4a.org

AARP
601 E. Street NW
Washington, DC 20049
1-888-687-2277
www.aarp.org

Alzheimer's Association
24 Hour Contact Center
for information, referral and support
800-272-3900
email:info@alz.org
www.alz.org

American Diabetes Association
1701 North Beauregard Street
Alexandria, VA 22311
1-800-DIABETES (1-800-342-2383)
AskADA@diabetes.org

Cancer Wellness Center, Northbrook, Illinois
Toll Free 1-866-292-9366
10847-509-9595

National Family Caregivers Association
10400 Connecticut Avenue, Suite 500
Kensington, MD 20895-3044
Phone: 301-942-6430
Fax: 301-942-2302
Email:info@thefamilycaregiver.org
www.thefamilycaregiver.org

National Alliance for Caregiving
4720 Montgomery Lane 5th Floor
Bethesda, MD 20814
Email:info@caregiving.org

Appendix

LIST OF EXERCISES

Printed in the United States
99344LV00001B/91-98/A